Neuroplasticity

How to Change Your Life by Changing Your Mind

(The Power of Positive Thinking and the Fascinating Ability of the Brain to Change Itself)

Thomas Farrell

Published By **Bengion Cosalas**

Thomas Farrell

Neuroplasticity: How to Change Your Life by Changing Your Mind (The Power of Positive Thinking and the Fascinating Ability of the Brain to Change Itself)

ISBN   978-0-9953324-5-4

No part of this guidebook shall be reproduced in any form without permission in writing from the publisher except in the case of brief quotations embodied in critical articles or reviews.

Legal & Disclaimer

The information contained in this book is not designed to replace or take the place of any form of medicine or professional medical advice. The information in this book has been provided for educational & entertainment purposes only.

The information contained in this book has been compiled from sources deemed reliable, and it is accurate to the best of the Author's knowledge; however, the Author cannot guarantee its accuracy and validity and cannot be held liable for any errors or omissions. Changes are periodically made to this book. You must consult your doctor or get professional medical advice before using any of the suggested remedies, techniques, or information in this book.

Table Of Contents

Chapter 1: Understanding Your Brain

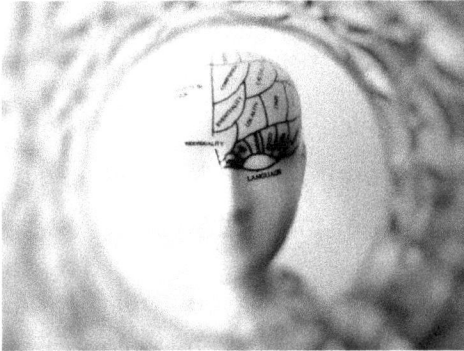

Understanding the thoughts is just like unraveling the mysteries of the universe, but in desire to peering into the cosmos, we are venturing inward. At its center, the human thoughts, the command middle of our frame, is a complicated community of billions of neurons talking thru trillions of connections referred to as synapses. This network isn't static but dynamic, normally reshaping and refining its connections. This outstanding capability is what we test with as neuroplasticity.

1.1What is Neuroplasticity?

Neuroplasticity, moreover called mind plasticity or neural plasticity, refers to the mind's capability to change and adapt due to revel in. It is derived from the words "neuron," which is probably the nerve cells within the brain, and "plasticity," implying changeability or malleability.

The mind engages in neuroplasticity inside the route of our lives in response to our environment, behaviors, wondering, emotions, and even in response to bodily damage. This technique lets in the neurons (nerve cells) in the mind to seize up on harm and sickness and to regulate their sports sports in reaction to new situations or to adjustments of their surroundings.

Neuroplasticity includes numerous one-of-a-type techniques that take location within the route of a person's lifetime. Many of these techniques involve synaptic plasticity, this is the ability of the synapses (the websites in which verbal exchange takes vicinity amongst neurons) to reinforce or weaken over the years. Changes in synaptic power may be brief-term (lasting a couple of minutes to numerous hours) or prolonged-term (lasting days to months or perhaps years), and this strengthening or weakening of synapses influences the mind's functionality to machine and take into account statistics.

Neuroplasticity gives the underlying foundation for lots of present day neuroscience, along facet our information of how we research, how we recollect, and the way our reports can shape us through the years. It has moreover extensively impacted our records of a way to treat positive neurological situations, collectively with stroke and stressful mind injury, in which recuperation procedures geared in the direction of harnessing the energy of neuroplasticity can help sufferers get better lost abilties.

In precis, neuroplasticity is the herbal mechanism with the aid of which we examine new things, shape recollections, adapt to new reviews, and get over thoughts accidents. It's a vital property of the mind that lets in us to continuously learn and adapt to an ever-converting international.

1.2 The Dynamic Brain

Historically, scientists believed that the mind, as soon as genuinely advanced, remained greater or less static at some point of maturity. However, over the last few a few years, groundbreaking research has established this notion to be some distance from the fact. Our brains, in desire to being everyday, are dynamic and ever-converting. This non-forestall capability to conform and exchange is underpinned thru the concept of neuroplasticity.

The human thoughts consists of approximately 86 billion neurons, every capable of making about 1,000 to ten,000 connections with different neurons. These connections form complicated networks that facilitate communication in the thoughts, making it viable for us to suppose, have a look at, take into account, understand, and execute movements. This as a substitute complicated community isn't stagnant; it's miles in a steady kingdom of flux, constantly forming and dissolving connections based totally on our testimonies, behaviors, and environment. This dynamic notable of the mind is what permits us to adapt and examine in the course of our lives.

When we've interplay in a brand new revel in or have a look at some element new, our mind responds by using strengthening the connections a number of the neurons worried in that method. This strengthening happens via a technique known as lengthy-time period potentiation, wherein the synapses (the tiny gaps in which indicators are handed among neurons) boom their efficiency. The extra regularly a selected synaptic pathway is activated, the more potent and further green the relationship turns into. This concept is often encapsulated with the resource of manner of the phrase "neurons that fireside together, cord collectively."

Conversely, whilst a neural pathway isn't always used, the connections weaken, and over the years, they may dissolve altogether. This technique, called synaptic pruning, ensures that our mind remains green, devoting resources only to the maximum regularly used and useful neural networks. This is the essence of the pronouncing "use it or lose it."

Our emotions, too, play a crucial function in shaping our mind's structure. Positive emotions can enhance neuroplasticity, improving the thoughts's capability to form new connections. On the opposite hand, persistent stress and terrible feelings can impair neuroplasticity, inhibiting the formation of recent neural pathways or maybe causing the shortage of present ones.

This ongoing dance of formation and dissolution, of strengthening and weakening, presentations the dynamic nature of our brains. Our thoughts, behaviors, research, and feelings aren't just merchandise of our brains—they may be the shapers of our brains. They sculpt the landscape of our minds, influencing our perceptions, our abilties, and in the end, our realities.

The information of our dynamic thoughts reveals an empowering reality: we aren't truly on the mercy of our neural wiring. With focused try and normal workout, we will harness the energy of neuroplasticity to adjust our neural pathways, reshape our brains, and trade our lives. This first rate capability to transform our brains gives us the machine to turn out to be architects of our non-public minds. In the chapters that observe, you may find out a way to wield the ones equipment to result in superb versions on your thoughts and your existence.

1.Three Neuroplasticity at Different Ages

The mind's functionality for trade isn't always uniform all through lifestyles. It varies at remarkable levels of improvement, from infancy to adulthood and into vintage age. Understanding how neuroplasticity operates across the ones ranges can provide crucial insights into our capability to research, adapt, and redecorate at any age.

Infancy and Early Childhood

During the early years of existence, the mind undergoes fast and profound changes. This period is marked by means of the use of a dramatic increase within the style of neural connections, a system referred to as synaptogenesis. Infants are born with all of the neurons they'll ever have, but those neurons are excellent partly stressed out. In the primary few years of lifestyles, the thoughts unexpectedly bureaucracy new connections, ensuing in a dense network of synapses.

At this degree, the mind is extensively plastic and receptive to reading. This heightened neuroplasticity allows children to take in new records brief and adapt to their environments. It's within the path of this time that foundational competencies like language, motor capabilities, and social abilities are received.

Adolescence

Adolescence marks each different vital duration in thoughts improvement. During this section, the mind undergoes large restructuring, mainly within the prefrontal cortex, this is responsible for complex cognitive abilities like decision making, impulse manage, and emotional regulation.

Simultaneously, the thoughts engages in synaptic pruning, a way in which unused or redundant neural connections are eliminated, making the thoughts more inexperienced. This section of severe mind remodeling can impact conduct, leading to the function impulsivity and emotional intensity of the teenage years.

Adulthood

In adulthood, neuroplasticity continues, albeit at a slower tempo in comparison to youngsters and childhood. The individual mind continues to be capable of forming new neural connections and analyzing new competencies. However, the price at which this takes place is predicated upon considerably on an person's way of life, stories, and habits.

Regular mental and physical stimulation, healthful nutritional conduct, proper sleep hygiene, and extremely good social interactions can all enhance neuroplasticity in adulthood, reinforcing the mind's capability for lifelong analyzing and model.

Old Age

Aging is frequently related to cognitive decline, but this does not suggest that the mind's functionality for exchange disappears completely. While positive cognitive competencies may additionally decline with age, different regions can also live robust or maybe beautify.

Even in antique age, the thoughts keeps so as to neuroplasticity. Learning new capabilities, preserving an energetic life-style, and appealing in everyday social interactions can assist hold or perhaps decorate cognitive characteristic in older adults, underscoring that our capacity for exchange extends at some point of our lifespan.

Neuroplasticity is a lifelong phenomenon. Though it can range at awesome levels of existence, the mind's potential to adapt and alternate stays all through our lifespan. Understanding this will empower us to harness neuroplasticity at any age, reinforcing the belief that it's miles in no way too past due—or too early—to alternate our brains and redecorate our lives.

1.Four The Power of Neuroplasticity

Neuroplasticity has added about a revolution in our information of the brain. The attention that our brain is malleable and capable of converting inside the path of our lives, no longer just in formative years, isn't something short of a paradigm shift. The implications of this electricity are far-accomplishing, impacting various domain names of our lives, collectively with getting to know, memory, healing from damage, intellectual health, and regular properly-being.

Learning and Memory

At the coronary heart of learning and reminiscence formation is the mind's plasticity. When we look at some thing new, our thoughts creates new neural pathways. As we keep to have interaction with that new facts or talent, the ones pathways are reinforced. For instance, whilst we research a new musical device, the mind office work new connections associated with hand-eye coordination, sound reputation, and emotional engagement with the song. With exercise, those connections decorate, and we come to be higher at playing the tool.

Similarly, our memories are saved in neural networks. Each time we recall a reminiscence, we're, in essence, visiting alongside that neural pathway. The greater often we revisit a memory, the stronger the pathway becomes, making it simpler to keep in mind that reminiscence in the destiny.

Recovery from Brain Injury

Neuroplasticity plays a vital role in recovery from thoughts damage. When a part of the mind is damaged due to damage or illness, superb elements of the thoughts can on occasion adapt and take over the out of place characteristic, a method known as purposeful reorganization. This functionality of the thoughts paperwork the idea of many rehabilitation treatments. For instance, in stroke rehabilitation, patients workout movements with the affected limbs to assist the mind rewire itself and regain manage over the ones movements.

Mental Health

The characteristic of neuroplasticity extends to highbrow health as properly. Many varieties of remedy, together with cognitive-behavioral treatment (CBT), are rooted in neuroplasticity. In CBT, sufferers studies to break terrible idea styles and replace them with more healthy ones, correctly rewiring the thoughts's response to sure triggers.

Research also indicates that practices like mindfulness and meditation can promote neuroplasticity, lowering stress and tension, improving interest and memory, and improving time-honored highbrow health.

Overall Well-being

Neuroplasticity affects no longer simply our cognitive talents and highbrow fitness but our common properly-being as properly. Healthy manner of existence conduct like ordinary physical exercising, a balanced weight loss program, and well sufficient sleep can all enhance neuroplasticity, important to superior cognitive function, decreased chance of neurodegenerative ailments, and higher highbrow health.

Chapter 2: The Myths And Facts Approximately

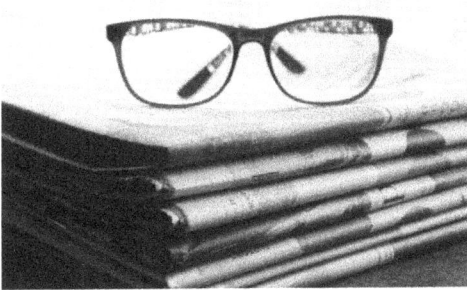

As our understanding of the mind and neuroplasticity has evolved, so have sure misconceptions approximately this complicated technique. While neuroplasticity has certainly transformative functionality, it is important to separate truth from fiction. In this bankruptcy, we are able to debunk a few commonplace myths approximately neuroplasticity and shed slight at the truth in the lower back of them.

Myth 1: Neuroplasticity best takes area throughout children

Fact: Neuroplasticity is indeed most active within the course of formative years, but it does no longer prevent after that. While it's miles proper that our brains make bigger and trade suddenly even as we're more younger, the thoughts keeps to form new neural connections and adjust gift ones all through our existence. This ongoing ability to change and adapt is essential to studying, memory, and healing from mind accidents.

The device can also sluggish down as we age, but it does not save you genuinely. Adults can and do take a look at new capabilities, adapt to new environments, or even recover from mind injuries or neurodegenerative illnesses, all manner to neuroplasticity. Even in antique age, sports activities inclusive of reading a present day language, gambling a musical tool, or engaging in physical workout can stimulate neuroplasticity and bring about extraordinary changes inside the thoughts's shape and characteristic.

So, the idea that the mind is only plastic for the duration of childhood is a fable. Neuroplasticity is a lifelong manner, and our brains stay able to getting to know and changing for the duration of our lives.

Myth 2: Neuroplasticity excellent applies to getting to know and memory

Fact: Neuroplasticity does play a vital feature in analyzing and reminiscence, but its impact is a notable deal broader. The technique of neuroplasticity underpins truly each component of our mind's characteristic in the course of our lifetime.

Neuroplasticity is vital not best for acquiring new information and skills however furthermore for forgetting irrelevant statistics, that could be a essential issue of healthy cognitive functioning. Moreover, it's miles pivotal in our functionality to conform to new environments or situations, in forming and retaining social bonds, and in preferred intellectual health.

In the context of mind accidents or diseases, neuroplasticity allows the thoughts to reorganize itself and catch up on broken regions. This functionality is the inspiration for healing and rehabilitation from conditions like stroke or traumatic thoughts accidents.

Even our emotions and thoughts can effect neuroplasticity. For instance, sustained stress or anxiety can purpose bad modifications in the thoughts, at the identical time as powerful feelings, mindfulness, and relaxation can decorate plasticity and sell trendy mind fitness.

So, at the equal time as neuroplasticity is essential to analyzing and memory, its importance extends to many special regions of mind characteristic and human revel in.

Myth three: Only great research and learning can exchange the thoughts

Fact: It's now not sincerely super memories or reading which could trade our brains; bad critiques also can cause substantial changes in our neural pathways.

For example, chronic pressure or trauma can result in numerous changes in the mind's shape and feature. Prolonged publicity to strain hormones, which encompass cortisol, can cause the hippocampus—a important area for learning and memory—to reduce. Similarly, experiencing trauma can purpose adjustments in the amygdala and prefrontal cortex, regions involved in emotional law and fear response, contributing to situations like positioned up-demanding stress sickness (PTSD).

Even repetitive awful wondering, a commonplace function of many intellectual health issues, can trade the thoughts. Over time, continual terrible concept patterns could make stronger the associated neural pathways, making those terrible belief styles greater effects brought about and extra tough to disrupt.

However, the mind's plasticity moreover gives wish for recuperation and restoration. Just as poor studies can purpose volatile changes, super critiques, healthful behaviors, and effective recovery interventions can sell useful mind adjustments. Practices like mindfulness, cognitive-behavioral remedy, and everyday physical interest can all foster excellent neuroplasticity, helping to restore and pork up neural pathways and improve highbrow fitness.

So, even as it's proper that our opinions and learning can alternate our mind, it's miles no longer only the superb ones which have an effect. However, the ability for neuroplasticity moreover method that bad changes aren't generally everlasting, and with the proper interventions, the brain can change for the better.

Myth 4: Neuroplasticity is continually beneficial

Fact: While neuroplasticity is crucial for our mind's capacity to analyze, adapt, and heal, it isn't always commonly useful. Sometimes, the adjustments that stand up in our thoughts can result in terrible outcomes. This concept is regularly called "maladaptive plasticity."

For instance, in sure neurological conditions like phantom limb syndrome, modifications within the thoughts can make a contribution to the persistence of ache or distinctive sensations from a limb that has been amputated. In this example, the mind's plasticity is not beneficial but rather ends in pain and distress.

Similarly, in the case of substance abuse and addiction, repeated exposure to addictive materials can motive adjustments inside the mind's reward tool. These modifications can manual connections among cues related to substance use and the desire to use the substance, making it hard to conquer addiction.

Another example is tinnitus, a scenario characterized through way of the belief of a constant ringing or noise within the ears.

Maladaptive plastic adjustments in the thoughts's auditory cortex can contribute to the continuation of these perceived sounds, even when there's no outside sound source.

So, while neuroplasticity is a effective and frequently effective aspect of thoughts feature, it isn't continuously beneficial. It can occasionally reason or contribute to problems, in particular at the same time as modifications inside the mind enhance negative or risky behaviors, sensations, or reviews. This is why information and effectively guiding our mind's plasticity can be so crucial for preserving and improving our fitness and properly-being.

Myth 5: Neuroplasticity way we can change our brains however we need

Fact: While neuroplasticity gives us the thrilling ability to shape and mold our mind's shape and function, there are truely limits to this malleability.

Firstly, our genetics play a function in putting certain parameters for thoughts improvement and characteristic. For example, on the identical time as we are in a position to investigate new languages at any age way to neuroplasticity, the capability for acquiring languages varies among human beings due in element to genetic versions.

Secondly, on the identical time as neuroplasticity can useful useful resource in recuperation from mind harm or disease, the amount of this recovery is usually recommended thru using the severity and location of the damage. Certain extreme thoughts injuries may additionally additionally additionally restriction the capability for beneficial restoration, notwithstanding the thoughts's plastic skills.

Thirdly, the diploma of plasticity varies all through the thoughts. Some areas of the thoughts, just like the hippocampus (worried in memory and mastering), display a immoderate degree of plasticity, on the equal time as others are a good deal a great deal much less changeable.

Lastly, age plays a function in neuroplasticity. While plasticity happens sooner or later of our lives, the fee of new neural connections formation and the functionality for tremendous reorganization of those connections decreases as we age.

Therefore, on the same time as neuroplasticity offers us with an extraordinary potential to research, adapt, and heal, it does not deliver us infinite manage to shape our mind but we need. Nevertheless, the adjustments we can have an effect on via our behavior, mind, and reviews are powerful and might extensively impact our cognitive capabilities, intellectual fitness, and ordinary first rate of lifestyles.

Chapter 3: The Relationship Amongst Habits, Thoughts,

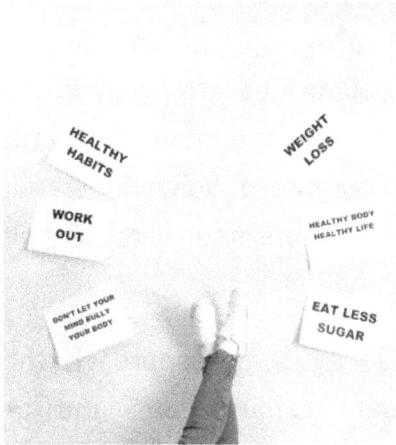

Neuroplasticity, the mind's capability to exchange and adapt, is a first-rate phenomenon that underlies masses of our lifestyles opinions. An critical detail of this plasticity revolves throughout the formation of habits and the character of our thoughts. How we act and anticipate on a ordinary basis can notably impact our thoughts's shape and feature.

3.1 Habits and Neuroplasticity

Habits are an integral a part of our lives, governing a whole lot of our every day movements from the immediately we awaken to whilst we go to sleep. From brushing our tooth to growing our morning espresso, conduct allow us to perform ordinary obligations with minimum intellectual effort. But how are those behavior standard, and what function does neuroplasticity play in this machine?

Neuroplasticity is the approach thru which our thoughts adjustments and adapts in reaction to enjoy. When we engage in an hobby time and again, the mind starts to bolster the neural pathways associated with that interest. The connection some of the neurons involved becomes extra inexperienced, permitting us to carry out the movement more rapid and with less conscious attempt.

This principle is encapsulated in a idea known as Hebb's Law, regularly simplified as "neurons that fireside together, wire together." The extra often a particular collection of neurons fires, the stronger the connections among them turn out to be. Over time, this collection of neuronal firing will become an increasing number of computerized, in the long run forming a addiction.

For example, allow's do not forget getting to know to stress a car. At first, each motion - from turning at the ignition to handling the guidance wheel, accelerator, and brakes - requires conscious belief and attempt. However, as we time and again exercising those moves, the neuronal connections associated with them turn out to be more potent. Over time, the ones movements come to be automatic, forming a dependancy, and we are able to strain without considering each step.

However, neuroplasticity is a double-edged sword. Just because it allows us to form useful conduct, it could furthermore reason the formation of risky behavior. For instance, if someone time and again makes use of a substance like alcohol or capsules, the thoughts strengthens the neural pathways related to the pride and praise skilled from the substance. This can result in a cycle of craving and use that characterizes addiction.

Understanding the characteristic of neuroplasticity in addiction formation gives effective insights into how we are able to alternate our behavior. By consciously choosing our actions and constantly training new behaviors, we are capable of harness the energy of neuroplasticity to create more healthy behavior. On the turn problem, expertise this method moreover permits us understand why breaking vintage conduct can be tough, because it calls for weakening properly-installed neural pathways.

In the give up, records neuroplasticity gives us a scientific basis for wish. Regardless of techniques ingrained our conduct is probably, our brains are capable of change. With consistency, staying energy, and the proper techniques, we're able to harness the energy of neuroplasticity to shape our conduct and our lives in beneficial techniques.

3.2 Thoughts and Neuroplasticity

Just as our movements can form our brains through the device of neuroplasticity, so also can our thoughts. The repetitive forms of thinking we interact in can substantially have an impact on the shape and function of our brains, impacting our highbrow and emotional nicely-being.

Every notion we have got triggers a unique sample of neural interest inner our brain. Each time we revisit a specific belief, the neural connections concerned in triggering that concept are reinforced, making it less complicated and extra computerized to cause the identical concept in the future. This is the idea of idea conduct, or habitual ways of thinking that grow to be ingrained through the years.

For example, if we regularly engage in self-critical thinking, the neural pathways associated with the ones terrible thoughts come to be stronger and extra computerized. Over time, this could purpose an improved tendency inside the path of self-complaint, decrease arrogance, and a higher danger of highbrow health problems like despair and anxiety.

On the other hand, often engaging in splendid questioning, which include expressing gratitude or training mindfulness, can decorate the neural pathways associated with the ones satisfactory thoughts. Over time, this may assist foster a greater effective thoughts-set, decorate vanity, and promote intellectual health.

This is not to mention that we ought to attempt to assume surely all of the time. After all, it is natural and healthy to revel in various feelings, together with terrible ones. However, facts the impact of our thoughts on our thoughts can encourage us to cultivate healthier idea patterns.

Just like changing our moves, changing our thoughts calls for conscious attempt and steady workout. Cognitive techniques which includes cognitive-behavioral treatment (CBT), mindfulness-primarily based definitely cognitive remedy (MBCT), and different mindfulness practices can be in particular effective in assisting us apprehend and modify our concept patterns, harnessing the energy of neuroplasticity to enhance our highbrow fitness.

So, the following time you find out your self caught in a cycle of horrible wondering, recollect: your thoughts have the electricity to form your brain. With staying power, exercising, and the right techniques, you can harness this strength to domesticate extra wholesome concept conduct and decorate your nicely-being.

3.3 Leveraging Neuroplasticity for Positive Change

Recognizing the strength of neuroplasticity offers us with a profound and transformative facts: our every day behavior and thoughts, whilst repeated constantly, can reshape our thoughts, in the long run changing our behaviors, emotions, and everyday highbrow well-being. This way we've got the capability to consciously direct adjustments in our mind to result in exceptional trade in our lives. Here are a few strategies to leverage the electricity of neuroplasticity effectively.

Cultivate Mindfulness:

Mindfulness includes maintaining a 2nd-to-moment cognizance of our mind, emotions, physical sensations, and the surrounding environment. By education mindfulness, we will take a look at our habits and mind without judgement, this is the first step in the direction of changing them. Mindfulness also can lessen strain, beautify emotional regulation, and promote immoderate incredible modifications within the thoughts.

Engage in Regular Physical Exercise:

Physical exercise promotes neuroplasticity through manner of stimulating the producing of neurochemicals and growth elements that decorate the fitness and growth of neurons. Regular physical exercise can decorate cognitive feature, lessen the chance of neurodegenerative diseases, and improve intellectual fitness.

Pursue Lifelong Learning:

Continuous studying and intellectual stimulation can decorate neuroplasticity, improve cognitive function, and put off cognitive decline as we age. This should encompass reading a new language, gambling a musical tool, or maybe taking on a new interest. The secret is to undertaking the mind to create and beautify new neural connections.

Practice Good Sleep Hygiene:

Sleep plays a vital function in reminiscence consolidation, a method this is predicated upon on neuroplasticity. Moreover, persistent sleep deprivation can impair cognitive characteristic and highbrow health. Maintaining awesome sleep hygiene can as a end result support healthful neuroplasticity.

Foster Positive Social Connections:

Positive social interactions can stimulate neuroplasticity and make contributions to improved cognitive feature and intellectual health. By keeping a supportive social network, we can harness the strength of neuroplasticity to enhance our common nicely-being.

Engage in Regular Meditation:

Meditation, like mindfulness, can bring about modifications within the mind that beautify severa components of cognition and intellectual fitness. Regular meditation can reduce stress, beautify interest and memory, and promote a popular revel in of nicely-being.

Chapter 4: Mindful Practices To Boost

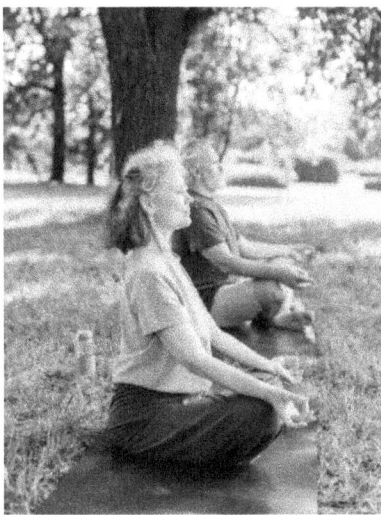

Neuroplasticity, our mind's capability to alternate and adapt, is shaped via our actions, thoughts, and critiques. One especially powerful way to harness neuroplasticity to improve our mental fitness and properly-being is thru mindfulness practices. Mindfulness encourages us to popularity on the triumphing 2d, selling a heightened consciousness of our mind, emotions, and sensations. In this bankruptcy, we will find out numerous mindful practices which could beautify neuroplasticity.

four.1 Mindfulness Meditation

Mindfulness meditation is a effective device that can help us harness the electricity of neuroplasticity. This exercising is centered on guiding our attention to the prevailing second and embracing it with out judgment. It's about listening to our mind, emotions, sensations, and the environment spherical us.

Here's the way to exercising mindfulness meditation:

Find a Quiet and Comfortable Place:

Start via locating a quiet spot in which you can sit down without disturbances for a while. This can be a devoted nook in your own home, a quiet park, or even your place of job in advance than or after your workday.

Choose Your Position:

Sit on a chair or a meditation cushion on the floor. The motive is to sit down down in a posture this is strong and strong, but additionally comfortable. Keep your again straight away, however now not stiff. Rest your palms to your knees or for your lap.

Focus on Your Breath:

Close your eyes gently and bring your interest in your breath. Feel the air because it enters and leaves your nostrils, the upward thrust and fall of your chest or stomach. Don't try to manage or alternate your breathing - without a doubt word it as it is.

Be Present:

As you attention on your breath, you can have a have a look at that your mind begins offevolved to wander, caught up in mind approximately the past or the destiny, or swept up in judgments or daydreams. This is in reality everyday and a part of the manner. When you be aware this taking location, lightly deliver your hobby once more for your breath without judging yourself.

Practice Regularly:

Aim for consistency in place of duration. Even a few minutes every day may want to make a massive distinction. Over time, you can discover that you may meditate for longer durations, however the secret is to installation a ordinary daily dependancy.

Mindfulness meditation can result in big changes inside the thoughts's shape and characteristic. Studies have mounted that everyday exercise can growth the density of gray rely in thoughts areas associated with reading, memory, emotion law, and empathy. It can also reduce interest in the "default mode network" - the part of the mind active in some unspecified time in the future of thoughts-wandering and related to ruminative, terrible mind.

By training mindfulness meditation regularly, we are capable of leverage the electricity of neuroplasticity to enhance our attention, lessen stress, control our emotions greater correctly, and enhance our common highbrow properly-being.

four.2 Body Scan Meditation

Body experiment meditation is a few other conscious exercising that may growth neuroplasticity and promote relaxation and self-reputation. This exercise entails systematically shifting your attention via particular factors of the frame, from the toes to the pinnacle of the pinnacle.

Here's the manner to exercising frame check meditation:

Choose Your Position:

This meditation is commonly finished lying down, however you could moreover do it sitting in a snug and robust feature. Ensure you are in an area in which you could continue to be quiet and undisturbed at some point of the exercise.

Begin with Deep Breathing:

Close your eyes and start through taking some deep, calming breaths. Inhale slowly, preserve for a second, and then exhale completely. As you try this, begin to be aware the feeling of your body mendacity (or sitting) and the sensation of your breath entering and leaving your frame.

Start the Body Scan:

After a couple of minutes, shift your interest in your body. You may begin at the toes, noticing any sensations gift. This might embody warmth, coolness, strain, tingling, or maybe no sensation in any respect. The key's to have a have a look at the sensations with out judgment.

Move Through Your Body:

Slowly flow into your interest up thru your frame - your ankles, calves, knees, thighs, pelvis, stomach, chest, lower back, shoulders, hands, palms, neck, face, and the pinnacle of your head. Spend a while at each location, noticing any sensations, tension, or relaxation.

Connect with Your Breath:

If your mind wanders off (that is honestly natural), lightly guide it returned to the subsequent a part of the body or be part of it collectively together with your breath. Don't rush; the intention is to move with steady recognition.

Conclude the Practice:

Once you have got scanned via your complete body, take a second to experience your body as an entire. Notice the way you revel in. Then, regularly convey movement lower returned into your body, stretch, and open your eyes.

Practicing body take a look at meditation can enhance hobby of our physical presence and help us revel in extra grounded. It has been associated with decreased strain and anxiety, higher hobby, advanced sleep, and everyday well-being. It is likewise used therapeutically in mindfulness-primarily based interventions, collectively with Mindfulness-Based Stress Reduction (MBSR), to alleviate pretty a few bodily and intellectual fitness signs and signs and signs. By mission practices like this, we will actively mold our brains to sell extra healthful forms of notion and behavior.

four.3 Mindful Eating

Mindful eating is a practice that engages our complete hobby at the method of eating, allowing us to have amusing with our meals, recognize our frame's starvation and fullness cues, and increase a more healthy dating with meals.

Here's the manner to exercise aware consuming:

Eliminate Distractions:

Turn off the TV, located away your cellular telephone, and try to consume in a peaceful and quiet surroundings. The purpose is to hobby your complete interest for your meal.

Appreciate Your Food:

Before you start eating, take a 2d to realize the food within the the the front of you. Consider the try that went into making ready it and the nutrients it's going to offer your frame.

Engage All Your Senses:

As you eat, examine the colours, textures, smells, sounds, and of direction, the flavors of your food. Try to find out terrific substances and spices.

Eat Slowly:

Take small bites and chunk very well. Eating slowly not nice permits you to have amusing with the flavors greater certainly, however moreover offers your frame the time it desires to method starvation and fullness cues.

Listen to Your Body:

Pay interest on your frame's starvation and fullness signs. Eat while you enjoy physical hungry, and forestall ingesting while you experience satisfied however now not overly complete.

Cultivate Gratitude:

After completing your meal, take a second to unique gratitude for the nourishment your meals gives.

Mindful consuming can transform our relationship with meals. It can assist us ruin loose from horrible eating behavior, lessen overeating, decorate our amusement of food, and enhance our digestion.

Neuroplastically talking, schooling aware consuming can create new, healthful neural pathways associated with eating and satiety, changing older, an awful lot a lot much less healthful conduct and responses. For example, it is able to assist damage the cycle of eating in response to emotional cues in preference to physical hunger.

In essence, with the beneficial useful resource of ingesting mindfully, we are capable of harness the power of neuroplasticity to sell a more healthful dating with food and decorate our regular nicely-being.

These are just a few of the numerous conscious practices that may decorate neuroplasticity. The secret's to find a exercising that resonates with you and make it a part of your every day recurring. Remember, consistency is essential in harnessing neuroplasticity. It's not approximately making large modifications abruptly but about small, steady efforts that add up over the years to create huge, lasting alternate on your brain and your lifestyles.

In the following chapters, we're able to discover more techniques to promote neuroplasticity, which include physical exercise, lifelong studying, and powerful social connections. By incorporating those numerous practices into your existence, you may leverage the power of neuroplasticity to decorate your highbrow health, cognitive talents, and ordinary well-being.

Chapter 5: Nutrition And Neuroplasticity

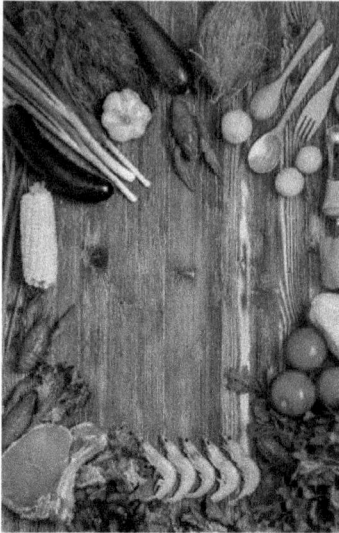

It's regularly stated that "you're what you eat," and that is specially real with regards to your thoughts. The food you consume can substantially have an effect at the health and functioning of your mind, which include the system of neuroplasticity. In this financial ruin, we are able to delve into the feature vitamins performs in neuroplasticity and find out how adopting a thoughts-wholesome food regimen can decorate your cognitive capabilities and giant properly-being.

5.1 The Role of Nutrition in Neuroplasticity

The meals we eat have a profound impact on our thoughts's fitness, improvement, and functioning. Nutrition substances the uncooked materials that the mind wants to carry out its severa obligations, which consist of neuroplasticity. In this segment, we can delve deeper into how particular vitamins can effect neuroplasticity and cognitive capabilities.

Omega-three Fatty Acids:

Omega-three fatty acids, specially DHA (Docosahexaenoic acid), are critical for mind fitness. They are a essential thing of neuronal mobile membranes, enhancing their fluidity and influencing receptor function. This supports the advent and protection of synaptic connections, a key aspect of neuroplasticity. Omega-3s additionally possess anti-inflammatory homes, which could shield the thoughts from damage and growing old.

Antioxidants:

Antioxidants, together with nutrients C and E, beta-carotene, and flavonoids, combat oxidative stress in the mind, a primary cause of neurodegenerative ailments. Oxidative pressure can impair neuroplasticity and cognitive function, so ingesting additives rich in antioxidants can assist protect the mind and decorate its plasticity.

B Vitamins:

B vitamins, specially B6, B9 (folate), and B12, are critical for brain fitness. They are worried in homocysteine metabolism, and excessive stages of homocysteine had been associated with an extended danger of neurodegenerative sicknesses. These vitamins moreover play a feature inside the manufacturing of neurotransmitters and the protection of the mind's structural integrity, influencing neuroplasticity.

Polyphenols:

Polyphenols are plant compounds with sturdy antioxidant and anti inflammatory results. They can decorate neuroplasticity via way of selling the boom of new neurons (neurogenesis) and protective cutting-edge neurons from damage. They can also furthermore improve conversation among neurons, assisting studying and memory.

Micronutrients:

Several distinctive micronutrients, together with iron, zinc, and magnesium, are involved in severa thoughts capabilities, which incorporates neurotransmission and neuroplasticity. They are critical for the everyday functioning of the thoughts and cognitive fitness.

Probiotics and Prebiotics:

Emerging research indicates that the intestine microbiota can effect thoughts feature and conduct, collectively with learning and memory, through the intestine-thoughts axis.

Probiotics (useful bacteria) and prebiotics (food that feed those micro organism) can resource a wholesome gut microbiota, which in turn may additionally beautify neuroplasticity.

In end, nutrients performs a crucial function in assisting neuroplasticity. The mind requires a constant deliver of precise vitamins to create and improve synaptic connections, generate new neurons, and hold the fitness of modern-day neurons. By eating a balanced, nutrient-dense weight loss program, we are able to provide our brains with the important building blocks to assist neuroplasticity and ordinary cognitive function.

five.2 Brain-Boosting Foods

Nutrition performs an important characteristic in our brain's health and function, which consist of our reminiscence, attention, and temper. Consuming super mind-boosting foods can enhance cognitive function and facilitate neuroplasticity. Let's dive into a number of those food which is probably regarded to be mainly beneficial for our brains:

Fatty Fish:

Fatty fish like salmon, trout, and sardines are wealthy assets of omega-3 fatty acids, particularly DHA and EPA. These fats are crucial for mind fitness, as they keep the fitness and characteristic of neurons, lessen contamination, and sell the boom of latest neurons and synaptic connections.

Blueberries:

Blueberries and one-of-a-kind deeply colored berries supply anthocyanins, a fixed of plant compounds with antioxidant and anti-inflammatory results. They remove mind aging and enhance memory, helping neuroplasticity.

Turmeric:

The active compound in turmeric, curcumin, has been verified to transport the blood-thoughts barrier and straight away blessings the brain. It has top notch antioxidant and anti-inflammatory blessings, boosts degrees of the thoughts hormone BDNF, which aids neuroplasticity and the increase of new mind cells.

Broccoli:

Broccoli is packed with antioxidants and food regimen K, seemed for helping thoughts health. The antioxidants in broccoli lessen infection and counteract oxidative pressure.

Pumpkin Seeds:

These seeds encompass a wealthy deliver of antioxidants that defend the body and mind from free radical harm. They're additionally an amazing supply of magnesium, iron, zinc, and copper, all critical for mind fitness.

Dark Chocolate:

Dark chocolate is filled with a few mind-boosting compounds, together with flavonoids, caffeine, and antioxidants. The flavonoids in chocolate accumulate inside the areas of the mind that deal with studying and reminiscence.

Oranges:

Oranges are a brilliant supply of vitamins C, this is prime for stopping highbrow decline. Consuming enough portions of weight loss program C-rich substances can guard in the direction of age-associated intellectual decline and Alzheimer's ailment.

Green Tea:

The caffeine and antioxidants determined in inexperienced tea can enhance brain characteristic, alongside side superior thoughts plasticity, brain growing old, mood, and memory.

Incorporating those thoughts-boosting components into your weight loss program can make a contribution substantially to retaining a healthful mind and promoting neuroplasticity. Eating a nutritionally balanced eating regimen whole of varied cease stop result, vegetables, lean proteins, and healthy fat can guide a healthy mind and empower the energy of neuroplasticity.

5.Three Balanced Diet and Hydration

A balanced diet and unique enough hydration are vital to everyday health and fitness, and they play a essential feature in cognitive function and thoughts fitness as nicely.

Balanced Diet

A balanced healthy dietweight-reduction plan offers all of the important vitamins our our bodies - and specially our brains - want to feature properly. A balanced weight loss program usually consists of:

Fruits and veggies: They are excessive in nutrients, minerals, and fiber, but low in calories. Try to devour quite a few amazing end result and veggies to get a huge range of vitamins.

Whole grains: Foods like oatmeal, brown rice, entire grain bread, and quinoa are exceptional sources of fiber and B vitamins.

Lean proteins: Fish, chicken, lean meats, beans, and nuts are actual belongings of awesome protein, it's essential for mind health.

Healthy fats: Foods like avocados, nuts, seeds, and fish are wealthy in healthy fat, which encompass omega-three fatty acids, which may be useful for thoughts fitness.

Dairy or dairy alternatives: These are an fantastic supply of calcium and food plan D.

Try to restriction your consumption of added sugars, salt, and dangerous fats. These can not best make contributions to physical health troubles but also can impact your mind fitness and cognitive characteristic.

Hydration

Staying hydrated is in reality as vital as consuming a balanced food regimen for keeping mind health. Water makes up approximately 75% of the mind and plays a vital function in mind characteristic. Dehydration can impair cognitive functions together with interest, reminiscence, and motor skills.

Here are a few suggestions to ensure you stay hydrated:

Try to drink at least 8 glasses of fluid steady with day. This can consist of water, tea, coffee, milk, and fruit juices. However, water is the tremendous preference as it's far calorie-unfastened and could now not contain any additives.

Eat masses of stop end result and greens. They are high in water content fabric material and make a contribution for your each day fluid consumption.

Carry a water bottle with you to encourage everyday eating.

Be privy to your frame's cues. Thirst, dry mouth, fatigue, and reduced urine output are symptoms and symptoms and signs and symptoms that you is probably dehydrated.

In quit, a balanced food regimen and proper hydration are key to promoting proper thoughts fitness and improving neuroplasticity. They offer the essential nutrients and hydration that our brains need to function optimally. As you navigate your journey to harness the power of neuroplasticity, keep those dietary recommendations at the primary facet to nourish and gasoline your thoughts.

five.Four The Gut-Brain Connection

The Gut-Brain Connection

The gut-thoughts connection is a bidirectional communique tool amongst our digestive tract and our mind. This gadget consists of the relevant concerned device, enteric frightened device (furthermore known as the "2nd brain" placed in our intestine), and the endocrine tool. It's an rising vicinity of take a look at that has captivating implications for know-how the hyperlink among our gut health and mind health.

The human intestine is domestic to trillions of bacteria together referred to as the gut microbiota. Research indicates that those microorganisms play a vital feature in our regular health, influencing the entirety from our digestion to our immune machine, and curiously, even our brain feature and intellectual health.

How Does the Gut Influence the Brain?

1. Neural Pathways: The gut and the thoughts are without delay related thru neural pathways, particularly the vagus nerve. The intestine can send signals to the mind via the ones nerve connections, influencing thoughts function and conduct.

2. Immune System: A giant part of the body's immune cells live within the intestine. When the steadiness of gut micro organism is disturbed, it could trigger an immune response that could have an effect on brain fitness and characteristic.

three. Hormones and Neurotransmitters: The gut micro organism also can have an effect on the brain via generating various bioactive substances, which includes neurotransmitters like serotonin and dopamine, and awesome chemical substances that have an effect on neural signaling and thoughts fitness.

Implications for Neuroplasticity

Emerging studies shows that the gut microbiota might also have an effect on neuroplasticity. Changes inside the composition of the intestine microbiota had been proven to have an effect on studying, reminiscence, and cognitive flexibility in animal models. While studies in humans continues to be in early degrees, it's miles recommended that a healthy and numerous gut microbiota want to probably guide neuroplasticity and cognitive characteristic.

Incorporating masses of fermented ingredients (like yogurt, kefir, sauerkraut, and kimchi) and excessive-fiber meals (like cease result, vegetables, legumes, and entire grains) to your healthy dietweight-reduction plan can sell a wholesome gut microbiota. Avoiding immoderate consumption of processed food, that could negatively effect intestine health, is likewise truely beneficial.

In end, the intestine-thoughts connection offers a captivating attitude on how our dietary picks can effect our mind health and neuroplasticity. By searching after our intestine fitness, we can be able to assist our mind fitness and harness the strength of neuroplasticity.

Chapter 6: Physical Exercise And Brain Health

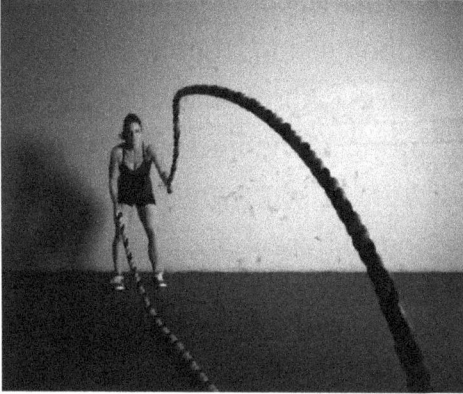

In this bankruptcy, we discover the vital link amongst bodily exercise and thoughts health, specially highlighting how normal bodily interest can enhance neuroplasticity, increase cognitive characteristic, and improve basic brain health.

6.1 The Benefits of Physical Exercise

Physical exercise has a huge range of benefits, from improving bodily fitness to enhancing cognitive feature and intellectual well being. Let's delve into those benefits:

1. Improved Cognitive Function: Regular physical workout has been demonstrated to enhance various components of cognitive function, which encompass interest, memory, vital questioning, and trouble-fixing skills. This takes place through the progressed manufacturing of neurotrophic elements (at the side of BDNF), which encourage the growth and differentiation of neurons and synapses.

2. Enhanced Mood: Exercise stimulates the release of endorphins, frequently called 'experience-suitable hormones'. Endorphins help to elevate mood, reduce strain, and offer a experience of health.

three. Reduced Risk of Chronic Disease: Regular physical activity can reduce the hazard of developing numerous chronic ailments, together with coronary heart ailment, stroke, kind 2 diabetes, and exceptional styles of most cancers. It can also help manage those conditions if they'll be already present.

four. Improved Sleep: Regular physical interest assist you to nod off faster and deepen your sleep. It additionally lets in to regularize the sleep-wake cycle, most important to extra constant, restful sleep.

five. Increased Energy Levels: While it would seem counterintuitive, everyday bodily exercising can actually decorate your electricity ranges. This takes vicinity as workout improves your frame's efficiency and staying strength, permitting you to do greater with a fantastic deal much less fatigue.

6. Better Weight Control: Regular physical hobby combined with a balanced food regimen can assist keep a wholesome weight or beneficial useful resource in weight reduction. This takes location as exercising will increase the charge at which your body burns calories.

7. Enhanced Neuroplasticity: Exercise stimulates the increase of new neural connections, improving neuroplasticity. It will also increase the size of the hippocampus, a

part of the mind vital for reminiscence and reading, primary to higher reminiscence typical overall performance.

eight. Delayed Cognitive Decline: Regular bodily workout has been associated with a do away with in the onset of cognitive decline and dementia. In human beings already diagnosed with Alzheimer's disorder, exercise can help to gradual the improvement of the infection.

In precis, bodily exercising is a effective device for preserving commonplace fitness and improving cognitive function. It's a cornerstone of a healthy manner of life and a powerful pleasant pal in the quest to harness the power of neuroplasticity.

6.2 Incorporating Physical Exercise into Your Daily Routine

Integrating physical hobby into your day by day routine can be a task, specially with the busy and regularly sedentary existence masses parents lead. However, with some planning and creativity, it's far in reality practicable. Here are a few suggestions:

1. Set Clear Goals: Set sensible and measurable goals for your self. They might be as clean as "walk for half-hour each day" or "attend yoga lessons in keeping with week". Having clear desires will offer you with a goal to aim for and make it a good deal much less complicated to track your improvement.

2. Choose Activities You Enjoy: You're more likely to paste to an exercising normal in case you experience the sports. Whether it's miles on foot, biking, swimming, dancing, yoga, or institution sports sports, pick out a few issue which you sit up straight for.

3. Make It a Habit: Try to exercising on the equal time every day, so it becomes part of your each day ordinary. It may be first issue in the morning, at some stage in a lunch break, or in the midnight after art work.

4. Break It Down: If you can not find out a prolonged non-stop time slot for workout,

ruin it down into shorter intervals. For instance, three 10-minute walks may be actually as effective as one 30-minute walk.

five. Use the Buddy System: Exercising with a chum or family member need to make the interest more fun, and you may encourage each unique to live heading inside the proper direction.

6. Use Technology: Fitness apps and wearable gadgets let you show your progress, provide feedback, and preserve you stimulated. They often have exercise mind and may be a wonderful tool for keeping consistency.

7. Be Active Throughout the Day: Look for strategies to feature extra bodily hobby in your ordinary day. Take the steps in preference to the elevator, park a bit in addition from your holiday spot and walk the relaxation of the manner, or have "on foot meetings" at art work.

8. Listen to Your Body: Rest is essential for restoration and stopping injuries. Incorporate

rest days to your exercising time table and in case you're feeling tired, opt for lighter sports activities sports like on foot or stretching.

Incorporating bodily workout into your every day recurring does now not require drastic adjustments. Start small, make it interesting, and be constant. Over time, the ones small steps can cause large enhancements for your bodily fitness, thoughts fitness, and great extremely good of existence.

Chapter 7: Sleep And Brain Plasticity

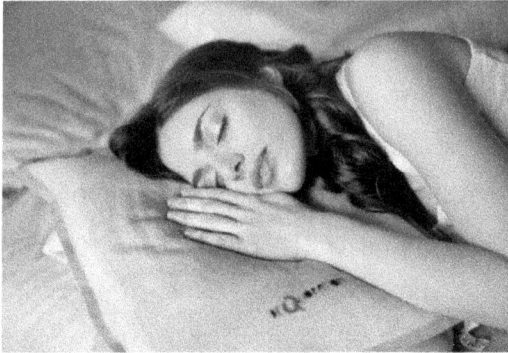

In this financial disaster, we delve into the charming dating among sleep and thoughts plasticity. We will find out the effect of sleep at the thoughts's capacity to exchange and adapt, and the way an first-rate night time's sleep can beautify our cognitive function and popular mind fitness.

7.1 The Role of Sleep in Brain Plasticity

Sleep is an vital a part of our lives that proper now affects our brain fitness. Beyond truly supporting our bodies recharge, it performs a critical feature within the consolidation of memory and learning, because of this selling mind plasticity. Here's a deeper check the location sleep plays in brain plasticity:

Memory Consolidation: During sleep, our brains are quite energetic. The studies we have had at a few diploma within the day are being processed and consolidated into long-term memories. This way essentially takes region throughout fast eye movement (REM) sleep, a degree of deep sleep in which we regularly dream. It's throughout this time that the neural connections that form our recollections are bolstered.

Synaptic Plasticity: Sleep additionally performs a essential position in synaptic plasticity – the ability of synapses to reinforce or weaken over the years. Synapses are the factors of verbal exchange among neurons, in which signs are transmitted. During sleep, the synapses that had been used intently at some point of the day get a threat to rest and get higher, preserving the stability of synaptic energy and supporting within the formation of new connections.

Neurogenesis: Emerging research shows that sleep also can support neurogenesis - the advent of new neurons. In specific, REM sleep appears to play a position within the maturation of those new cells, mainly inside the hippocampus, an area of the mind crucial for memory and mastering.

Brain Cleansing: While we sleep, our mind moreover undergoes a kind of 'housecleaning'. The glymphatic tool, the brain's specific waste clearance device, becomes greater active within the path of sleep. It flushes out waste merchandise that have gathered inside the thoughts in the course of our waking hours, together with beta-amyloid, a protein associated with Alzheimer's sickness. This cleaning system enables hold most desirable thoughts function.

Emotional Regulation: Sleep also performs a massive position in regulating our feelings. During REM sleep, our brain strategies emotional information, which enables us reply efficiently to emotional stimuli at the same time as we are wide unsleeping.

In conclusion, sleep performs a essential characteristic in promoting thoughts plasticity. It allows reminiscence consolidation, aids in synaptic plasticity and neurogenesis, permits cleanse the thoughts, and plays a function in emotional law. Ensuring appropriate enough and high-quality sleep is an essential detail of harnessing the strength of neuroplasticity.

7.2 Improving Sleep for Better Brain Health

Getting an incredible night time time time's sleep is crucial for mind fitness and harnessing the electricity of neuroplasticity. Here are a few techniques to improve your sleep:

Establish a Sleep Schedule: Consistency is pinnacle close to sleep. Try to visit mattress and wake up on the identical time every day, even on weekends. This facilitates regulate your body's inner clock and may make falling asleep and waking up less complicated.

Create a Restful Environment: Your dozing surroundings plays a crucial function in determining how nicely you sleep. Keep your room dark, quiet, and at a cushty temperature. Consider using earplugs, a nap mask, or a white noise device if desired. Make positive your bed and pillows are cushty and supportive.

Limit Screen Time Before Bed: The blue slight emitted through video show devices on smartphones, capsules, computer systems, and TVs can interfere together together with your frame's manufacturing of melatonin, a hormone that regulates sleep. Try to reveal off the ones devices at least an hour earlier than bedtime.

Pay Attention to What You Eat and Drink: Avoid large food, caffeine, and alcohol near bedtime. These can disrupt your sleep or purpose you to rouse in the middle of the night.

Incorporate Physical Activity into Your Day: Regular bodily pastime permit you to doze off quicker and deepen your sleep. However, avoid energetic workout close to bedtime as it would intervene together collectively along with your sleep.

Manage Stress: High levels of strain or anxiety can intervene together with your sleep. Techniques which includes meditation, deep respiratory, or yoga will let you lighten up and control pressure, principal to higher sleep.

Seek Professional Help if Needed: If you have got were given continual troubles with sleep, searching for scientific advice. Sleep problems which incorporates sleep apnea and insomnia are treatable, and addressing those situations can considerably enhance your sleep and, consequently, your mind health.

Remember, improving sleep isn't always generally a brief restore however a gradual way that includes modifications on your life-style and conduct. However, the advantages on your cognitive function and ordinary mind fitness make it nicely well worth the attempt. Sleep well to harness the power of neuroplasticity virtually!

The Role of Emotional Health

In this bankruptcy, we find out the feature of emotional health in brain plasticity and common cognitive feature. Emotional fitness refers to our capacity to recognize and manipulate our emotions. It's a important detail of our well-being and has a huge effect on our mind fitness.

eight.1 Understanding Emotional Health

Emotional fitness is a critical a part of our widespread properly-being and is honestly as vital as our bodily health. It involves our ability to govern and specific the feelings that stand up from the u.S.A.And downs of existence. However, being emotionally healthful isn't in reality equated to the absence of bad feelings. Instead, it's miles approximately having the ability to surely be given and precise those emotions in a wholesome manner, being able to deal with annoying situations, and getting better from life's setbacks.

A strong basis in emotional fitness furthermore allows us to forge robust relationships, make accurate options, and maintain a pleasing outlook. Here are a few key additives of emotional fitness:

Emotional Awareness: This includes recognizing your private emotions and those of others. It's step one within the direction of knowledge your emotional reactions to existence's reviews.

Emotional Regulation: Emotional health includes the capability to reply to emotions in a suitable way. This doesn't imply avoiding bad feelings, but as an alternative understanding them and coping with them in a manner it's far optimistic instead of detrimental.

Resilience: Life is complete of disturbing conditions. Emotional health includes the capability to get better from adversity, trauma, and strain. This resilience is built over the years as we discover ways to face challenges and navigate emotional ache.

Autonomy: Emotionally healthy humans have a enjoy of manipulate over their lives and can make selections for themselves. They revel in confident in their capacity to form their very private lifestyles conditions.

Self-esteem: A wholesome revel in of vanity is a vital part of emotional fitness. When you price yourself and function right vanity, you sense consistent and worthwhile and feature commonly terrific relationships with others.

Empathy: The potential to apprehend and percentage the feelings of others is a key element of emotional fitness. Empathy allows us to build connections with others, that is vital for our social properly-being.

Understanding our emotional health and mastering the manner to nurture it may substantially beautify our lives, relationships, or maybe our bodily health. Emotional health is not constant. Just like our brains, it's miles something that we are able to alternate and decorate over time. We will later see how it's miles cautiously tied to the concept of neuroplasticity.

eight.2 Emotional Health and Brain Plasticity

Our emotional health and mind plasticity are intrinsically related, with each influencing and affecting the opportunity. Here's a better have a observe their connection:

Emotion Regulation and Brain Function: Our brains play a critical feature in emotion law. The prefrontal cortex, especially the ventromedial and dorsolateral regions, artwork with the amygdala, a key player in our emotional responses, to assist us observe and respond to emotional situations. These interactions shape neural pathways that may be strengthened or altered through neuroplastic techniques. Thus, our critiques, in particular emotionally charged ones, can form those pathways and effect our emotional regulation.

Stress and Brain Plasticity: Chronic strain can be destructive to each our emotional health and mind plasticity. Stress hormones, like cortisol, can impair neurogenesis (introduction of new neurons) and synaptic plasticity, particularly in the hippocampus, a area essential for memory and getting to know. Conversely, strain management strategies can promote thoughts plasticity and resilience, improving our potential to deal with stress.

Positive Emotions and Brain Health: Positive emotions were established to stimulate the discharge of neurotransmitters like dopamine and serotonin, which not most effective make us feel suitable but furthermore stimulate neuroplasticity. Positive intellectual states and sports activities alongside facet happiness, gratitude, mindfulness, and meditation can beautify mind plasticity through strengthening current neural connections and promoting the formation of new ones.

Negative Emotions and Brain Health: Similarly, bad emotions also can leave their mark on our brains. Chronic anxiety, depression, and extended publicity to pressure can bring about unfavorable changes within the mind shape and characteristic. These adjustments could have an impact on areas just like the prefrontal cortex and the amygdala, which might be essential for emotion law and response.

Trauma and Brain Plasticity: Traumatic recollections can considerably effect the thoughts. They can reason changes in areas associated with memory, emotion regulation, and strain response. Understanding this may assist us admire the significance of mental interventions, like psychotherapy, in assisting to mitigate the terrible effect of trauma.

Healing and Brain Plasticity: Emotional recovery strategies, like treatment, meditation, or even the system of having vintage, can assist rewire the thoughts in more wholesome approaches. This issue of neuroplasticity offers desire for emotional and mental healing and the capacity for boom and trade, regardless of our past.

In essence, our emotional research, each first rate and bad, play a massive characteristic in shaping our brains. Understanding this connection can assist us leverage the power of neuroplasticity to beautify our emotional health and well-known nicely-being.

8.Three Promoting Emotional Health for Brain Health

Enhancing emotional fitness isn't always virtually beneficial to your mental nicely-being; it may moreover decorate your thoughts health thru the energy of neuroplasticity.

Chapter 8: 30-Day Action Plan For Brain Transformation

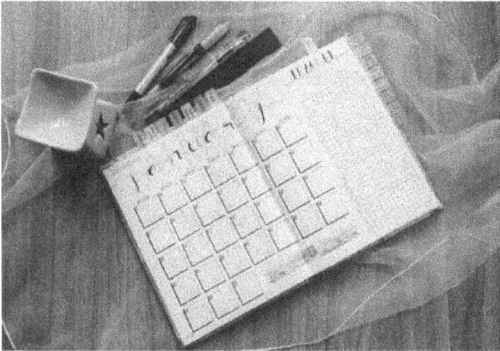

After information the strength of neuroplasticity and its ties to our behavior, mind, nutrients, physical workout, sleep, and emotional health, we are able to now delve into the realistic trouble of our journey: a complete 30-day motion plan designed to harness the power of neuroplasticity and redecorate your thoughts for higher.

This plan is designed to help you progressively incorporate lifestyle modifications that promote neuroplasticity. Remember, every person's journey is particular, so revel in free to regulate this plan to higher healthful your dreams and conditions. Let's get started out!

9.1 Week 1: Building Awareness

The first step inside the path of creating any full-size exchange is to extend a easy interest of what desires to trade. This week is all approximately paying hobby, noticing our present patterns, and laying the concept for the transformation we choice.

Day 1-three: Start a Mindfulness Meditation Practice

Begin with mindfulness meditation. Set aside five mins every day for quiet reflection. Find a relaxed and comfortable region in which you could sit down undisturbed. Focus to your breath, the upward push and fall of your chest, the sensation of the air coming into and leaving your nostrils. If your thoughts begins offevolved to wander, gently guide your recognition lower returned on your breath. As you workout this, you are not only reducing strain and selling relaxation, however you are moreover schooling your mind to recognition and be present. Gradually boom the period of your meditation instructions as you get comfortable with the procedure.

Day four-5: Keep a Journal of Your Habits

Habits shape our lives more than we frequently recognise. For the ones two days, keep a magazine noting your every day conduct. These may be as smooth as your morning espresso normal or as complex as your paintings patterns. Pay hobby to the triggers that provoke those behavior, the moves you're taking, and the rewards you get from them. Understanding this loop let you later on the same time as you want to modify or introduce new behavior.

Day 6-7: Incorporate Brain-Boosting Foods into Your Diet

Nutrition plays a essential function in thoughts health. For those two days, attention on adding greater thoughts-boosting components into your diet. Include greater surrender result and vegetables, which can be full of antioxidants which can defend your mind. Incorporate lean proteins like chook, turkey, or fish, which give amino acids important for neurotransmitter production. Stay hydrated, as even moderate dehydration can have an effect on cognitive feature. These initial steps in nutritional adjustments will lay the foundation for a greater complete dietary plan later on.

Building interest takes time, so be affected person with yourself in the course of this week. It's approximately gathering statistics and information your self better, now not approximately making large modifications proper away. Remember, the adventure of 1 thousand miles starts offevolved offevolved with a single step.

9.2 Week 2: Establishing New Habits

Now that we have advanced a extra consciousness of our modern patterns, it's time to start putting in new conduct that sell mind fitness. Remember, habits take time to form and grow to be computerized, so be patient with your self as you navigate this phase.

Day eight-10: Add a Simple Exercise Routine to Your Day

Physical exercise is vital for mind fitness. It promotes the increase of recent neurons and permits within the formation of latest neural connections. Begin via incorporating a clean workout ordinary into your day. This may be a brisk walk inside the morning, a yoga consultation, or any physical hobby which you enjoy. Starting with some component you want will increase the possibility that you can stick with it. Over time, try to purpose for as a minimum half-hour of moderate exercise maximum days of the week.

Day 11-12: Practice Mindful Eating

Eating is an interest that we frequently do mindlessly, however it offers a exceptional opportunity to exercising mindfulness. For the ones   days, take some time to devour your food with out distractions. Savor the flavor, texture, and scent of your food. Pay interest to your frame's starvation and fullness cues. Mindful ingesting can decorate your entertainment of food, assist prevent overeating, and promote a more fit courting with meals.

Day thirteen-14: Implement a Sleep Routine

Sleep is critical for mind fitness. It's a time while your thoughts consolidates memories, clears out waste products, and rejuvenates itself. Implement a nap everyday that lets in you get 7-nine hours of super sleep every night time. This should possibly incorporate putting a ordinary sleep and wake time, developing a calming pre-bedtime habitual, and making sure your sleep surroundings is dark, quiet, and cool.

Establishing new conduct is a gadget of trial and errors. Not everything will art work flawlessly the first time, and this is ok. The secret's to be chronic and affected individual, and to have a very good time your improvement along the manner. Remember, it is the small, regular changes that result in large changes through the years.

nine.3 Week three: Strengthening Emotional Health

This week, we turn our attention to our emotional health. Our feelings and feelings are not virtually abstract entities, they've a profound impact on our thoughts characteristic and ordinary well-being. By nurturing our emotional health, we're able to further beautify our thoughts's neuroplasticity and potential for trade.

Day 15-17: Keep a Gratitude Journal

Gratitude has effective outcomes on our mind. It can growth our tiers of happiness, reduce stress, or maybe decorate our mind's capability to form new connections. For the ones 3 days, keep a gratitude mag. Each day, write down 3 stuff you're grateful for. They may be as large or as small as you want - the key is to in fact sense the gratitude as you write them down.

Day 18-19: Practice Stress Management Techniques

Chronic pressure can prevent neuroplasticity and negatively impact our brain fitness. Therefore, finding healthful approaches to control pressure is critical. This can also additionally need to involve deep respiratory sports, progressive muscle rest, yoga, or any hobby that permits you lighten up and unwind. Experiment with one-of-a-kind techniques and find what works notable for you.

Day 20-21: Nurture Your Relationships

Our relationships and social interactions can stimulate our brains and help us manipulate stress, thereby selling emotional health and neuroplasticity. Spend exceptional time with your family, reconnect with a chum you have not talked to in a while, or even interact in social activities that you enjoy.

Remember, emotional fitness is a crucial a part of common nicely-being, and with the aid of nurturing it, we are able to considerably enhance our mind's capability for trade. Be affected person with yourself, and take into account that emotional increase is a adventure, not a holiday spot.

nine.Four Week 4: Integrating and Enhancing

In this very last week of our plan, we aim to combine all the practices we've got been walking on and decorate them. By now, you've got started out to installation new behavior, have a clearer statistics of your patterns, and characteristic taken important steps to boost your mind's fitness. Now, it is time to tie the entirety collectively and take it to the next degree.

Day 22-24: Increase the Duration of Your Mindfulness Practice

By now, mindfulness must be turning into a regular part of your every day regular. During the ones 3 days, purpose to growth the period of your mindfulness exercising. Also, begin incorporating mindfulness into ordinary sports activities. This is probably as smooth as paying attention to your breath at the equal time as you're geared up in line, noticing the texture of water for your pores and skin on the equal time as you wash your palms, or being without a doubt gift whilst speaking to a pal.

Day 25-26: Evaluate and Replace Detrimental Habits

With your attention of your conduct now clearer, it is time to begin making significant adjustments. Identify conduct that is probably horrible for your brain health or everyday well-being. This will be excessive intake of alcohol, spending too much time on digital gadgets, or eating an excessive amount of processed meals. Begin to update those detrimental behavior with useful ones. Remember, that is a manner, so start with one dependancy at a time.

Chapter 9: Sustaining Change And Overcoming Challenges

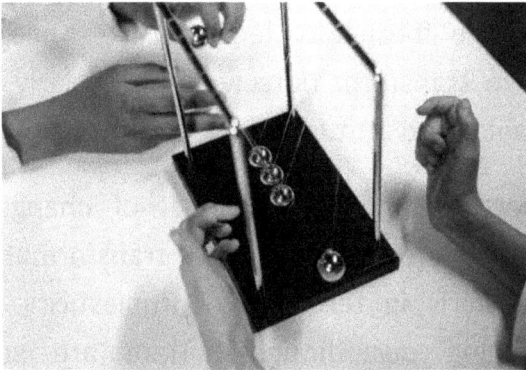

As you technique the prevent of your 30-day thoughts transformation journey, it's miles critical to look ahead and plan for the instances to go back. Changing your mind isn't always most effective a one-month task; it is a lifelong dedication to non-prevent growth and improvement. This bankruptcy will provide steering on maintaining the exceptional adjustments you've got got made and overcoming any challenges you may face within the destiny.

10.1 Understanding the Nature of Change

Change is an inherent a part of existence. From the seasons moving to the cells in our frame renewing, trade is ubiquitous. Yet, notwithstanding its pervasive nature, exchange frequently feels elusive while we aim to transform ourselves, particularly our behavior and attitude.

Understanding the individual of change is essential for a success transformation, particularly in terms of neuroplasticity and reshaping our thoughts. Here are some important factors to preserve in mind:

Change is Non-linear: Many people envisage change as a at once line, wherein development takes place in an instantaneous, uninterrupted collection. However, the fact is a long manner from this. Change is usually a non-linear approach, full of advances, retreats, and stagnation durations. You ought to probable discover which you make big development in the first few days of a state-of-the-art regular, simplest to discover yourself falling back into vintage behavior in line with week later. This is definitely everyday. Recognizing the non-linear nature of change permit you to be affected character with yourself and stay dedicated although development seems slow or non-existent.

Change Requires Repetition: Your thoughts loves repetition. It is thru everyday repetition that neural pathways grow to be stronger and conduct become ingrained. Just as a river often carves a deep valley, repetitive thoughts and behaviors over the years create robust neural networks in our mind. Hence, to enact lasting alternate, you need to be organized to replicate new mind, behaviors, and sports activities activities time and again once more until they grow to be part of who you are.

Change Involves Discomfort: Change, via its very nature, pushes us out of our consolation zones. You should in all likelihood revel in ache or resistance whilst in search of to alter your physical sports, mind, or behaviors. This is due to the truth your mind is stressed out to decide on familiarity and safety. However, stepping out of your consolation zone is vital for increase and transformation. Recognizing and accepting this pain can also want to make it much less complicated with a view to encompass alternate.

Understanding the individual of alternate can substantially increase your chances of a fulfillment transformation. So, as you hold on your adventure to harness the electricity of neuroplasticity, preserve those elements in mind. They will assist you hold a practical mindset, live affected person with your self, and persevere on your quest to transform your thoughts and existence.

10.2 Strategies for Sustaining Change

Once you have got got started the journey of trade, the following task is retaining it. Change can regularly revel in exhilarating on the start at the same time as motivation is immoderate. However, retaining those modifications over the long time may be more difficult, particularly even as the initial burst of motivation starts to vanish. Here are some techniques that assist you to hold change:

Consistency Over Intensity: It's easy to start with high depth whilst motivation is at its top. But it's miles consistency, now not depth, that results in lasting exchange. Focus on making small, consistent adjustments that you can preserve always in location of making drastic adjustments that may be difficult to keep.

Set SMART Goals: Specific, Measurable, Achievable, Relevant, and Time-certain (SMART) desires can offer a easy direction in advance and make it a good deal much less hard in case you want to track your development. Remember, small, incremental desires are frequently extra powerful than massive, daunting ones.

Incorporate Changes into Your Daily Routine: The handiest manner to keep change is to make it a part of your ordinary lifestyles. This should recommend incorporating mindfulness into your each day adventure, making equipped a mind-wholesome meal as a part of your normal weight-reduction plan, or inclusive of a couple of minutes of physical activity into your ordinary damage time.

Cultivate a Growth Mindset: A boom thoughts-set, as coined by using psychologist Carol Dweck, is the notion that capabilities and intelligence may be evolved via dedication and tough artwork. When you have were given a growth mindset, you notice traumatic conditions as possibilities to have a look at and increase, in preference to obstacles.

Celebrate Your Progress: Change is hard artwork and it's miles crucial to renowned your development, irrespective of how small it would appear. Celebrating your achievements can decorate your motivation and self warranty, making it much less complex which will preserve trade.

Seek Support: Having a help network may need to make a exceptional difference. This may be a friend or family member who's also making changes, a professional train or therapist, or maybe a supportive community, each offline or on line.

Remember, retaining alternate is a journey. There may be times whilst you could stumble or veer astray. But, with these strategies in your toolkit, you'll be higher prepared to live on course and make lasting adjustments that harness the strength of neuroplasticity.

10.Three Overcoming Challenges

In the path to self-development and change, going via annoying conditions is inevitable. From wavering motivation to surprising obstacles, the road can regularly seem riddled with hurdles. Yet, the crucial component to lasting trade lies not in retaining off those stressful conditions, however in mastering to overcome them. Here are a few techniques that can help you navigate those limitations:

Anticipate and Plan for Challenges: The first step in overcoming disturbing situations is looking ahead to them. Are there precise triggers or conditions that make it tough to paste for your new conduct? Once you choose out those capability stumbling blocks, you may create a plan to address them. This may want to in all likelihood suggest finding a exercise friend to keep you accountable, making ready thoughts-wholesome food earlier to keep away from risky consuming, or setting a bedtime alarm to make certain you get enough sleep.

Adopt a Problem-Solving Mindset: When you encounter a task, as opposed to viewing it as a setback, address it as a hassle to be solved. This shift in mind-set may want to make traumatic conditions a good deal less daunting and further ability. Break down the problem into smaller additives and address them one after the alternative.

Be Flexible and Adaptive: Sometimes, notwithstanding our incredible plans, topics do not exercising the way we count on. In such times, being bendy and adaptive can assist. If a specific strategy isn't running, be open to attempting something one of a kind. Remember, the goal isn't always to stick rigidly to a plan, however to find what works high-quality for you.

Practice Self-Compassion: It's herbal to sense aggravated or disheartened on the identical time as faced with worrying conditions. But beating your self up may want to make it even tougher to triumph over those hurdles. Instead, exercise self-compassion. Acknowledge that everybody faces stressful conditions and makes mistakes, and address yourself with the identical kindness and statistics you could expand to a friend.

Cultivate Resilience: Resilience is the functionality to bounce back from adversity. Cultivating resilience allow you to navigate stressful situations and come out stronger at the alternative facet. This would possibly contain developing a robust resource community, working closer to mindfulness and self-care, or studying to reframe terrible mind.

Overcoming demanding situations is a crucial part of the journey closer to lasting change. These strategies will equip you with the gadget you need to navigate hurdles, making it tons much less difficult as a manner to harness the strength of neuroplasticity and rework your lifestyles.

Remember that the power to trade your mind and redesign your existence is inner you. It's a adventure, now not a vacation spot. As you continue to harness the energy of neuroplasticity, you may now not only enhance your thoughts health but moreover beautify your regular exceptional of lifestyles. Keep shifting in advance, remain curious, and keep to nurture your thoughts. The journey inside the direction of a greater in form, greater colorful brain is one that lasts an entire life. Embrace it, and enjoy the journey.

Chapter 10: Stories Of Transformation

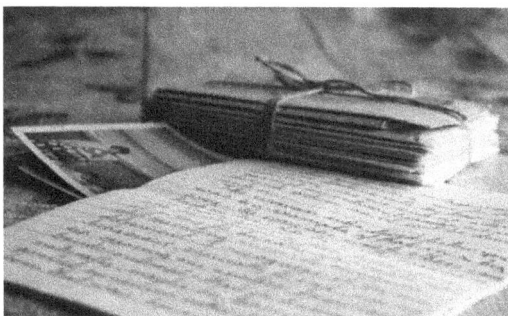

One of the most inspiring elements of neuroplasticity is its capability to facilitate real, tangible transformation. As we draw close to the surrender of this ebook, we flip our interest to numerous individuals who've harnessed the power of neuroplasticity to convert their lives. These stories feature inspirational reminders of what's possible at the identical time as we determine to trade and put in force the necessities said in this ebook.

11.1 Story of Jake: From Sedentary to Active

Jake, a 35-yr-vintage software program program application developer, spent maximum of his day sitting within the the front of a computer. His task required prolonged hours, which precipitated a sedentary way of lifestyles, awful nutritional conduct, and minimum bodily hobby. Over the years, he determined weight advantage, skilled continual decrease lower back pain, and felt constantly worn-out. He knew he had to make a alternate, but he did not recognize wherein to begin. The project of remodeling his manner of existence regarded overwhelming, daunting.

After stumbling upon the concept of neuroplasticity, Jake felt a glimmer of want. The concept that he ought to rewire his brain to crave physical hobby in preference to dreading it felt empowering. With this newfound expertise, he determined to make bigger a plan, integrating the standards of neuroplasticity to assist him transition from a sedentary lifestyle to an active one.

In the primary week, he focused on building interest, which involved expertise his present day conduct and figuring out possibilities for change. Jake mentioned the instances he modified into maximum inactive and started out to introduce small bouts of physical interest. Instead of taking the elevator, he started out the usage of the stairs. During lunch breaks, he opted for quick walks across the block rather than surfing the net.

In the second one week, he took it a step further. Jake commenced out putting unique, measurable, possible, applicable, and time-sure (SMART) desires. He aimed to engage in slight-intensity exercise for as a minimum half-hour a day, five days in step with week. He started with the useful resource of incorporating brief taking walks durations into his every day walks.

By the 1/3 week, Jake located himself searching ahead to his exercise periods. He added range to his habitual, regarding sports activities like cycling and swimming, which helped him live engaged and brought approximately. He furthermore started out practising mindfulness at some stage in his exercising instructions, focusing on the rhythm of his breath and the sensation of his frame moving, making his exercises a meditative experience.

By the fourth week, exercise had emerge as an important a part of Jake's life. He located a big bargain in his back pain, had extra electricity within the course of the day, or perhaps began losing weight. He grow to be surprised to discover that he became not dragging himself to workout – instead, he found joy and success in being energetic. It become a smooth manifestation of neuroplasticity in movement.

Jake's adventure indicates us that even deeply ingrained conduct like a sedentary lifestyle may be modified via way of the usage of harnessing the electricity of neuroplasticity. It did not appear in a unmarried day, but with steady try, a clean plan, and a boom thoughts-set, Jake was capable of rewire his brain to no longer surely include but moreover experience bodily interest. His tale serves as an notion and proof of the transformative energy of neuroplasticity.

11.2 Story of Lisa: Overcoming Stress and Anxiety

Lisa end up an finished government at a chief tech enterprise. Although her career become a success, she often decided herself coping with high stages of strain and tension. She battled persistent insomnia, a constantly racing mind, and the incapacity to revel in her downtime because of continual worry. Recognizing that this became no longer a sustainable way to live, Lisa sought assist.

After reading about neuroplasticity, Lisa grow to be intrigued via the use of the concept of reprogramming her thoughts to better deal with stress. Guided with the useful resource of this idea, she decided to domesticate mindfulness practices to assist her manipulate anxiety.

In the primary week of her adventure, Lisa's number one recognition turn out to be on developing popularity of her pressure triggers and notion patterns. She started out to be conscious that her anxiety frequently peaked during immoderate-stakes meetings or even as handling tight cut-off dates.

In the second week, Lisa determined to position into impact a each day mindfulness meditation exercising. She commenced out with genuinely 5 minutes consistent with day, that specialize in her breath and searching at her thoughts without judgment. With everyday exercising, she observed a sluggish shift in her reaction to demanding situations—she changed into becoming lots much less reactive and greater targeted.

During the 1/3 week, Lisa prolonged her mindfulness workout beyond meditation. She made a aware attempt to be found in each 2nd, whether or not or not or now not she become consuming, the use of, or spending time together together with her own family.

This smooth workout helped her reduce the normal feeling of speeding and brought a sense of calmness to her existence.

By the fourth week, Lisa felt a extremely good exchange in her ordinary tension levels. She turn out to be sound asleep better, her mind become clearer, and he or she or he need to navigate traumatic conditions greater correctly. Furthermore, her relationships advanced as she have end up more gift and engaged.

However, Lisa knew that this changed into in reality the begin of her adventure. She understood that neuroplasticity is a lifelong technique and continued to commit effort and time to her mindfulness exercise, even after seeing upgrades.

Lisa's story demonstrates that thru harnessing the energy of neuroplasticity, we are capable of trade how we respond to stress and tension. Through constant mindfulness practices, she modified into capable of rewire her thoughts, lessen anxiety, and dramatically improve her super of life. This shows that no matter how ingrained our responses to pressure may be, with time, staying energy, and staying strength, trade is viable.

eleven.Three Story of Maria: Changing Dietary Habits

Maria have become a hectic mother of 3. Juggling her pastime, the kid's college schedules, and own family chores left her with little time or energy to reputation on her nutrients. She often discovered herself accomplishing for comfort meals and emotionally consuming to govern stress. Although she became well aware of the requirements of wholesome consuming, breaking free from the cycle of terrible dietary behavior seemed near impossible.

When Maria determined approximately neuroplasticity, she determined out that she can also need to probable exchange her courting with food. With a newfound want and determination, she determined to embark on a journey to undertake more healthy consuming behavior.

In the number one week, Maria centered on gaining attention of her present day ingesting behavior. She said down the whole lot she ate and began identifying styles. She determined out that she often skipped breakfast, snacked on excessive-sugar food for quick energy in the route of the afternoon slump, and overate within the evenings.

During the second one week, Maria commenced making small however impactful adjustments. She started out every day with a nutritious breakfast, which helped manage her electricity degrees more successfully at some degree in the day. She additionally began making geared up healthy snacks in advance to deal with the afternoon stoop with out resorting to sugary meals.

By the 1/3 week, Maria started experimenting with mindful eating. She made a conscious attempt to consume with out distractions, bite her meals very well, and truely have fun with every chew. This exercising helped her experience extra satisfied after food and averted overeating.

In the fourth week, Maria located sizeable changes. She had more strength, her garments in form higher, and he or she or he or he had fewer cravings for unstable meals. Most importantly, she began out playing the technique of getting equipped and eating healthy food.

Maria's journey demonstrates that neuroplasticity also can observe to our dietary behavior. It wasn't easy, and it required constant attempt to staying power. But over the years, Maria come to be capable of rewire her mind to crave nutritious substances in desire to terrible ones. Her tale shows that regardless of how lengthy we've had been given been caught in volatile patterns, exchange is possible via the strength of neuroplasticity.

eleven.4 Story of Tom: Healing from Trauma

Tom come to be a army veteran who had served in a warfare region. After he lower returned domestic, he suffered from publish-disturbing pressure disease (PTSD). He end up haunted with the useful resource of vivid reminiscences of battle, skilled flashbacks, and had troubles connecting emotionally along with his family and friends. Although he become physical consistent at domestic, his thoughts modified into even though trapped within the battlefield.

When Tom came in some unspecified time in the future of the idea of neuroplasticity, he realized that there is probably a manner to heal from his trauma. Inspired via the concept that he may additionally need to rewire his mind and trade his idea styles, Tom started out a adventure inside the direction of restoration.

During the number one week, Tom targeted on spotting his triggers and records his emotional responses. He observed that first-rate sounds, snap shots, or perhaps smells must right away shipping him back to the conflict vicinity, triggering a panic assault or emotional numbness.

In the second week, Tom began out a guided trauma-centered therapy that blanketed cognitive-behavioral techniques and mindfulness. This remedy aimed to assist him confront and reframe his disturbing recollections. He commenced to exercising grounding techniques to manipulate his tension and flashbacks.

By the 0.33 week, Tom started out out to introduce a each day meditation ordinary. He would possibly attention on his breath and exercise mindfulness, step by step growing his functionality to live present and decrease instances of flashbacks.

Chapter 11: How Our Thoughts Advanced

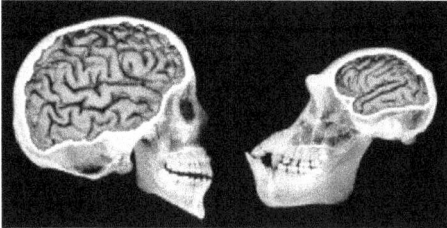

Throughout evolution, the human thoughts have long beyond thru massive changes. Initially, human beings had a small braincase, followed through way of sturdy jaws that facilitated consuming raw meals. However, with the invention of fireside, there was a marked change. The cranial difficulty improved in period, on the same time due to the fact the mandibles reduced, which allowed a more improvement of intelligence.

This anatomical evolution delivered blessings, as it freed the fingers from the movement of taking walks, permitting people to start the usage of gadget and manipulating the herbal environment in innovative strategies. As time handed, the cerebral cortex, answerable for complicated cognitive talents, also stepped forward in quantity. This growth supplied extra information processing thru perception and language.

These anatomical and cognitive modifications added with them the want for socialization. As human societies advanced, living capabilities and social corporation have come to be essential for collective development. Communication competencies and the formation of social bonds have grow to be critical factors for model and survival.

Thus, through the years, the human thoughts has developed remarkably. From a constrained cranial structure, we had been capable of expand an more and more state-of-the-art intelligence. The acquisition of manual talents, the boom of the cerebral cortex and social evolution were important additives on this evolutionary device, presenting us with the functionality to suppose, talk and collaborate in complicated methods.

Discovering Neuroplasticity

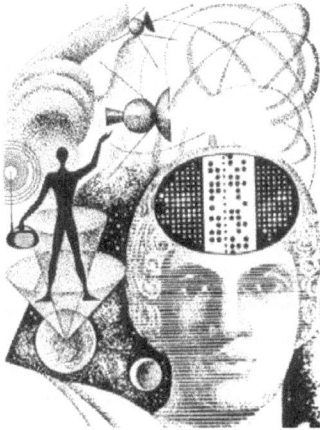

Neuroplasticity is a phenomenon that well-knownshows the brain's splendid functionality to conform and exchange all through existence. In the beyond, it changed into believed that the thoughts end up a static entity, with its neural connections fixed from start. However, contemporary studies have validated that this is not actual.

Neuroplasticity refers to the mind's potential to reorganize its synaptic connections, shape new neural pathways, and regulate its shape in response to environmental stimuli, tales, learning, and harm. This potential to trade and adapt is vital for cognitive improvement, getting better skills after mind injuries, and enhancing highbrow standard common performance.

The mind is made of billions of nerve cells known as neurons, which communicate thru synapses. These synapses are the connections between neurons and are liable for transmitting information in the brain. Through neuroplasticity, the ones synapses can be reinforced, weakened or perhaps created and eliminated.

There are essential sorts of neuroplasticity: structural plasticity and useful plasticity. Structural plasticity includes bodily changes in the structure of the thoughts, which incorporates the increase of recent neurons, the formation of dendrites and the introduction of latest synaptic connections. Functional plasticity, rather, refers to changes in neural hobby and inside the conversation pathways amongst neurons.

Neuroplasticity happens thru severa mechanisms. One of the precept ones is the functionality to enhance or weaken synapses, known as synaptic potentiation or synaptic melancholy, respectively. These approaches are stimulated via the repetition, depth and significance of the stimuli acquired with the useful aid of the brain.

In addition, neuroplasticity is likewise stricken by factors along side the environment, emotion, physical workout, food and learning. Stimulating the thoughts through cognitive challenges, meditation practices, physical hobby and a healthful diet can sell neuroplasticity and enhance mind development.

This is critical for maximizing the mind's capacity and overcoming barriers. By expertise that the mind can change, adapt, and expand at some point of existence, we can discover strategies and techniques that benefit our cognitive increase, harm recuperation, and highbrow properly-being.

The Fundamentals of the Brain: Understanding its shape and functioning

The human thoughts is a super organ, a wonder of nature that still intrigues scientists and researchers.

Its complexity and processing electricity are truly amazing. To recognize neuroplasticity, it is crucial to find out the basics of the mind, data its shape and the complicated functioning that makes it able to acting the most various cognitive and behavioral abilities.

The thoughts is split into numerous areas, every with particular capabilities. The outer layer of the mind is called the cerebral cortex and is liable for a number of the higher cognitive talents. It is break up into considered one among a kind areas which includes the frontal, parietal, temporal and occipital cortex, each with high-quality roles in perception, memory, language, motor manipulate and choice-making.

Beneath the cerebral cortex, we find deeper structures along aspect the hippocampus, the amygdala and the brainstem.

These structures play crucial roles in emotional processing, memory formation, sleep law, control of coronary coronary coronary heart and breathing rhythms, among one of a kind critical capabilities for the functioning of the organism.

Neurons are the important cells of the thoughts. They are chargeable for transmitting information via electrical impulses and chemical substances called neurotransmitters. Neurons connect to every extraordinary forming complicated and interconnected networks, permitting conversation and data processing inside the thoughts.

These connections amongst neurons are called synapses. Synapses are factors of touch among neurons wherein electric powered indicators are converted into chemical signs and vice versa. It is thru the synapses that facts is transmitted and processed, permitting the mind to feature as a sophisticated community.

Synaptic plasticity is one of the essential mechanisms involved in neuroplasticity. It refers to the capability of synapses to alternate their electricity and performance in transmitting information. When severe and repeated interest takes place in a neural circuit, the synapses in that circuit can decorate, making verbal exchange among neurons greater green. This phenomenon is known as synaptic potentiation.

Furthermore, the thoughts is fairly adaptable and can reorganize its connections in reaction to modifications in the environment, studying reviews and accidents. This capability to reorganize and form new synaptic connections is what makes neuroplasticity possible.

By unlocking the mysteries of mind shape and synaptic functioning, we are able to increase techniques and interventions that promote neural plasticity, boosting cognitive improvement, recuperation from mind harm and superior highbrow performance.

Flexible Brain: Unlock Your Potential with Neuroplasticity

If you could release your thoughts's full capability, what may additionally want to you have got got the capacity to carry out?

Imagine gaining know-how of new talents with out problem, overcoming challenges with agility, and accomplishing a degree of average performance you in no way idea feasible. It's all viable with neuroplasticity - the thoughts's first rate electricity to evolve, change and reshape itself.

The human thoughts is sort of a sponge thirsty for statistics and studies, and neuroplasticity is the important component to unlocking that capability. It permits us to reshape our thoughts, strengthening synapses, forming new connections and enhancing our highbrow ordinary overall performance.

With neuroplasticity, you could have a have a look at something from a modern language to playing a musical device. You can enlarge social skills, improve your memory, boom your creativity and increase your capability to treatment complicated troubles. There are no limits to what your flexible thoughts can benefit.

Imagine how transformative it might be if you can conquer fears and phobias, liberating your self from the shackles that save you you from dwelling genuinely. With neuroplasticity, you may rewire your thoughts, converting poor patterns with splendid ones, reaching a resilient and confident attitude.

Neuroplasticity is not handiest for the younger set. Your thoughts has the potential to conform and trade throughout your entire existence. No count your age, you could experience the benefits of neuroplasticity to enhance your super of lifestyles and reap your right potential.

So how will you liberate the strength of neuroplasticity?

Stimulate yourself with new demanding situations: Expose yourself to new opinions, examine high-quality abilties and constantly mission your mind. Try sports activities that stimulate splendid cognitive regions, at the side of puzzles, method games, mastering a modern musical device, or gambling a recreation.

Exercise your brain: Just much like the frame, the mind moreover dreams exercising to bolster itself. Dedicate time each day to sports sports that stimulate the thoughts, which consist of analyzing, writing, fixing math troubles, memory video video games and crossword puzzles. Stay mentally lively and challenged.

Practice non-prevent mastering: Never forestall mastering! Stay up to date on topics that hobby you and discover areas that pique your hobby. Learn a latest language, have a observe a brand new problem, take on line guides or attend workshops. Constant learning continues your thoughts continuously lively and encourages neuroplasticity.

Take care of your conventional health: A wholesome manner of life is critical for most green thoughts function. Make fine you eat a balanced weight loss plan rich in vital mind nutrients like omega-3s, vitamins and antioxidants. Exercise frequently, get sufficient sleep, and manage strain.

Explore meditation and mindfulness techniques: Meditation and mindfulness had been mounted to have incredible consequences on neuroplasticity. Take a few minutes each day to exercise meditation, focusing in your breath and the prevailing 2d. This enables to calm the thoughts, reduce stress and promote the formation of recent neural connections.

Stay Socially Connected: Interacting with others is a wonderful manner to stimulate your mind and sell neuroplasticity. Stay socially lively, be a part of groups, get involved in community sports activities, and domesticate vast relationships. Exchanging studies and sharing expertise make a contribution to mind boom.

Be regular and chronic: Neuroplasticity takes time and exercise. Be regular to your technique and stay with it although results aren't on the spot. Remember that each new experience and venture is an possibility to reshape your mind and achieve lasting outcomes.

By following this practical technique, you'll be growing a good environment to decorate your neuroplasticity and liberate your mind energy. Remember that each little motion counts and which you have the electricity to form your non-public mind.

Beyond Limits: The Neuroplasticity Revolution

The neuroplasticity revolution has been a milestone in expertise the human mind and its brilliant talents.

One of the maximum surprising discoveries about neuroplasticity is that it happens the least bit stages of life. From early thoughts development in adolescence thru maturity and antique age, our brains are constantly remodeling. This technique we will analyze and adapt in the direction of our adventure, difficult previously set up limits.

Brain plasticity can be determined at special levels. At a microscopic degree, synapses, which can be the connections among neurons, can be bolstered or weakened based totally on sorts of neuronal hobby.

New synapses can shape, permitting the advent of new neural circuits. This synaptic flexibility performs a key role in reading and reminiscence formation.

Furthermore, neuroplasticity can also be determined at a macroscopic degree, related to changes inside the organisation and form of the mind. Studies have showed that the in depth workout of sure capabilities can bring about structural changes, which incorporates an increase inside the length of precise regions of the mind associated with that capability. For example, professional musicians have structural modifications in mind areas worried in musical belief and motor coordination.

The neuroplasticity revolution has remarkable implications in hundreds of regions. In the world of rehabilitation, for example, expertise the mind's capability to transform itself after neurological accidents offers desire for those seeking out to get better out of place characteristic. Therapies based totally on neuroplasticity have been advanced to assist human beings with strokes, spinal twine accidents and distinct neurological situations.

Not to mention that neuroplasticity has implications in the vicinity of education. Understanding how the mind adapts and learns can assist boom more powerful educational procedures that bear in mind the uniqueness of every pupil and sell an surroundings conducive to intellectual growth.

The neuroplasticity revolution shows us that we are able to going past the boundaries that had been formerly imposed on us. Our thoughts has an brilliant functionality for model and growth, and it's far as a good deal as us to explore and make the maximum of this capability.

Chapter 12: The Connections That Drive Communication In The Brain

When we think about how the thoughts works, synapses play a key characteristic in transmitting facts amongst neurons. These small structures are chargeable for boosting conversation and the change of electrical and chemical indicators in the mind. Let's delve deeper into the captivating international of synapses.

A synapse is a specialized connection among two neurons wherein facts is transferred from one neuron to a few specific. It includes 3 foremost components: the presynaptic terminal, the synaptic cleft, and the postsynaptic terminal. These systems paintings collectively to ensure efficient communication between neurons.

The presynaptic terminal is the a part of the neuron that sends the electric sign. When an electrical impulse reaches the presynaptic terminal, it triggers the discharge of neurotransmitters, which might be chemical substances accountable for transmitting the sign to the following neuron. Neurotransmitters are saved in vesicles inside the presynaptic terminal and are launched into the synaptic cleft.

The synaptic cleft is the microscopic location among the presynaptic terminal and the postsynaptic terminal. It is in this vicinity that the transfer of neurotransmitters happens. This vicinity is vital for communique amongst neurons, as neurotransmitters should skip it to acquire the following neuron.

At the postsynaptic terminal, the obtained chemical sign is transformed decrease again into an electrical sign. Here, neurotransmitters bind to particular receptors gift on the membrane of the postsynaptic neuron. This connection triggers a chain of electrical sports activities that permit the propagation of the signal through the neuron and the continuity of the transmission of facts.

Synapses are fantastically dynamic and are constantly adapting and converting. Synapse energy, called synaptic plasticity, may be extended or weakened based totally on styles of neuronal interest. This synaptic plasticity plays a vital characteristic in studying and reminiscence formation, allowing connections amongst neurons to reinforce or weaken primarily based at the frequency and intensity of stimuli.

Synapses are chargeable for the mind's first-rate capability to technique facts, analyze, take into account, and carry out a myriad of complex skills. They form an complicated community of neuronal communication, allowing the thoughts to function as a specially coordinated device.

Understanding how synapses work is vital to know-how the complexity of the human mind and the diverse neurological conditions that may arise at the same time as synapses are dysfunctional. Ongoing studies are ongoing to in addition release the secrets and techniques and strategies of synapses and their impact on our cognition and conduct.

The Myths of Brain Capacity: Debunking Common Misconceptions

Over the years, many myths and misconceptions have emerged regarding human thoughts potential. These misconceptions can cause constrained facts or even underestimation of the mind's actual competencies. Let's debunk some of those myths and discover the fact inside the lower returned of brain electricity.

Myth: We simplest use 10% of our mind.

Truth: This well-known notion that we pleasant use 10% of our thoughts is a fable. In reality, the human thoughts is specially energetic and all its areas have specific competencies. Every a part of the mind plays an crucial function in our cognitive and behavioral functioning.

Myth: The mind does now not exchange after accomplishing adulthood.

Truth: Another not unusual false impression is that the mind stops converting and growing after adulthood. However, neuroplasticity, the mind's ability to conform and redesign, continues at some stage in life. The brain can form new connections, enhance synapses and adapt to new studies and analyzing at any age.

Myth: Our capabilities are determined with the aid of genetics and can not be changed.

Truth: While genetics play a feature in identifying positive mind developments, thoughts capacity goes beyond genetics. Brain plasticity allows us to accumulate new competencies, observe and enhance over the years. With right training, it's miles feasible to increase our abilties and attain better ranges of performance.

Myth: Men's and girls's brains are essentially taken into consideration one of a type.

Truth: While there are thoughts variations between men and women in terms of period and business enterprise, those variations do no longer recommend superiority or inferiority. Brain capability isn't always determined via gender, however as an possibility with the beneficial useful resource of the complex aggregate of genetic, environmental and person elements.

Myth: Intelligence is regular and can't be changed.

Truth: Intelligence is not a difficult and fast function. Studies display that intelligence can be evolved and superior during life. The mind has the capability to create new connections, deliver a boost to synapses and enhance your cognitive capabilities. Continuous analyzing and intellectual demanding situations can beautify the improvement of intelligence.

Debunking these myths is essential to data our thoughts's real capability. Our thoughts capacities are not restrained or static, but fluid and moldable.

Neurogenesis: The Formation of New Neurons

For a long term, it changed into believed that the formation of latest neurons, additionally called neurogenesis, end up a device certainly one of a kind to embryonic development and did not arise in maturity. However, modern-day research has found that the adult thoughts has the capability to generate new neurons in superb areas, a cute and fascinating phenomenon.

Adult neurogenesis takes region commonly in areas of the mind: the hippocampus and the olfactory bulb. The hippocampus plays an essential function in reading and reminiscence formation, whilst the olfactory bulb is worried in processing heady scent. These regions are in particular receptive to the formation of recent neurons because of their immoderate plasticity.

The technique of neurogenesis starts offevolved with neural stem cells, additionally known as neural progenitor cells. These cells have the capability to divide and differentiate into useful neurons. They are gift mainly regions of the brain, which include the subventricular vicinity of the olfactory bulb and the subgranular region of the hippocampus.

Adult neurogenesis is going through numerous levels. First, neural stem cells divide to deliver progenitor cells, that have the capacity to grow to be neurons. These progenitor cells then undergo a differentiation manner, wherein they collect the structural and realistic trends of mature neurons. Eventually, the newly normal neurons migrate to their suitable positions and set up synaptic connections with different contemporary neurons.

Adult neurogenesis is endorsed through using numerous elements. Regular physical interest, adequate sleep, enriched environment and stimulating learning are a number of the factors that sell the formation of latest neurons. Positive stimuli, together with emotionally big tales and cognitive disturbing conditions, can also enhance neurogenesis.

The importance of person neurogenesis lies in the truth that the formation of new neurons contributes to thoughts plasticity, the mind's potential to conform and change sooner or later of lifestyles. This functionality to generate new neurons offers the possibility to reshape neural circuits, improve present connections, and sell analyzing and memory formation.

In quick, adult neurogenesis demanding situations the belief that the formation of latest neurons is restricted to embryonic development. Our mind has the capability to regenerate and renew itself at some point of lifestyles, starting up thrilling opportunities for facts mind functioning and developing new recovery tactics. Neurogenesis is a powerful reminder that the mind is a remarkably dynamic and adaptable organ.

Chapter 13: The Pit Method

Have you ever puzzled how some humans have notable reminiscences, able to recollect minute information and keep statistics impressively? The solution may moreover lie in neuroplasticity, the brain's functionality to transform and adapt. And now, an thrilling and scientifically based totally completely approach has emerged as a effective device for growing high-quality reminiscence: the PIT Method.

PIT, which stands for "Planning, Intensity and Training", is a technique that makes use of the requirements of neuroplasticity to improve memory. Let's find out how every problem of the PIT Method plays a key function in this manner.

Planning: The first step to developing an terrific memory is strategic making plans. Identify what records is essential and worth remembering. Set clean dreams and goals for what you need to memorize. This will assist aim your efforts efficiently and optimize your reminiscence retention capability.

Intensity: Intensity is the key to boosting neuroplasticity. The more you've got interplay with the records you want to recall, the greater deeply it'll probable be processed and stored via the mind. Apply attention and attention techniques at the same time as studying. Create superb and emotionally appealing establishments to the information, as this can increase the chance that you can bear in mind it later.

Training: Just as an athlete trains to decorate his overall performance, reminiscence additionally requires systematic education. Dedicate time regularly to exercise your reminiscence. This can be completed via spaced repetition practices, periodic evaluations, and retrieval attempting out. These sports pork up neural synapses, consolidate records into prolonged-time period reminiscence, and growth your capacity to don't forget correctly.

In addition to the PIT Method, different complementary techniques can in addition extend the results. Using mnemonic techniques, along side acronyms, seen establishments and mind palaces, can increase your memory competencies. Practicing ordinary bodily exercise, healthy consuming and properly extraordinary sleep are also key to keeping a mind in amazing strolling order and promoting neuroplasticity.

Remember that neuroplasticity is not an at once technique. It requires consistency, staying power and staying strength. As you devote your self to the PIT Method and take a proactive method to reminiscence improvement, your thoughts will regularly reply, strengthening your mnemonic skills through the years.

So get prepared to challenge your limits, discover your thoughts's functionality and hold close the captivating international of memory. With the PIT Method and neuroplasticity for your component, you are on your way to reaching great reminiscence and starting off doorways to deep expertise and a sharp mind.

Neuroplasticity and Emotions: Transforming Negative Emotional Patterns

Emotions play a key feature in our lives, influencing our mind, behaviors and simple well-being. However, we will frequently get stuck in negative emotional styles that save you us from accomplishing emotional balance and happiness. The amazing statistics is that neuroplasticity, the mind's capability to transform and adapt, offers a powerful way to transform these patterns and domesticate extra fantastic, extra wholesome feelings.

The brain is a totally bendy and dynamic organ, able to reorganizing its neural connections in reaction to the reviews and stimuli we enjoy. This capacity for structural trade is the concept of neuroplasticity and allows us to actively form our emotional patterns.

Understanding the neural foundation of emotions

Emotions are complicated methods that include precise neural networks in our mind. The limbic device, which incorporates structures which incorporates the hippocampus, amygdala and prefrontal cortex, performs a key characteristic in regulating feelings. These structures artwork together to method, interpret, and respond to emotional stimuli.

When we over and over enjoy negative feelings, together with anxiety, fear, or unhappiness, the neural circuits associated with the ones emotions enhance and come to be extra resultseasily activated. This creates an ingrained emotional sample that may be hard to trade. However, neuroplasticity offers the opportunity to break out of these styles and create new, more healthy neural pathways.

Practicing emotional self-law

Emotional self-law is the ability to apprehend, recognize and modify our feelings in a healthy manner. It performs a important role in reworking terrible emotional patterns. Here are a few strategies which could assist:

a) Mindfulness: The workout of mindfulness lets in us to check our emotions without judgment, growing a extra popularity of the triumphing 2nd. By cultivating mindfulness, we're able to apprehend and take shipping of our terrible feelings with out getting carried away by way of the usage of them. This offers us the opportunity to respond consciously and constructively, in place of reacting mechanically.

b) Cognitive restructuring: Our emotional patterns are frequently rooted in horrible and distorted idea patterns. Cognitive restructuring consists of identifying and hard those bad thinking patterns, converting them with more realistic and pleasant thoughts. By wondering our proscribing ideals and adopting extra healthful perspectives, we're

143

able to rewire our brains for a extra balanced emotional reaction.

c) Stress regulation: Chronic strain has a giant effect on our feelings. Finding powerful techniques to control pressure, collectively with regular workout, relaxation strategies, adequate sleep and fitness care, is critical for transforming awful emotional patterns. By reducing strain, we create an environment conducive to neuroplasticity and the formation of recent exceptional neural connections.

Gradual and stable publicity to emotions

To redecorate horrible emotional patterns, it is essential to step by step display your self to tough emotions, but in a safe and managed way. This may be executed through publicity remedy or through practices consisting of healing writing, wherein we specific our feelings thru writing.

Chapter 14: Cultivating Wonderful Feelings

In addition to remodeling terrible emotional styles, neuroplasticity moreover permits us to domesticate high-quality feelings. By directing our interest and motive within the direction of top notch research, we will beef up the neural pathways related to the ones feelings.

Practices like gratitude, cultivating kindness, and appreciating the triumphing can help reshape our brains for added emotional resilience and lasting happiness. The extra we've interaction in awesome emotions, the greater the mind adapts and creates new neural connections that preference these emotional states.

In brief, neuroplasticity gives us the possibility to convert horrific emotional patterns and domesticate more balanced emotional fitness. By education emotional self-regulation, step by step exposing ourselves to hard emotions, and cultivating high-quality emotions, we are capable of actively reshape our brains and pave the manner for a fuller, greater high-quality emotional lifestyles. Remember that transformation takes time, practice and perseverance, but the outcomes are genuinely worth it. Harness the strength of neuroplasticity to create lasting exchange in your emotions and experience a more emotionally healthful and pleasing life.

regenerative plasticity

This form of plasticity is in particular evident in peripheral nerves, which may be placed out of doors the mind and spinal cord.

When a peripheral nerve is injured, because of an twist of fate or trauma, as an instance, regenerative plasticity can arise. This way that broken axons have the capability to boom another time, reconnecting to tissues and organs that have been damaged. This regeneration is a sluggish technique and might require the supervision of healthcare specialists to make sure proper restoration.

However, it's far essential to spotlight that now not all peripheral nerve injuries are mission to complete regeneration. In a few instances, while the harm can be very severe and impacts the supporting shape of the nerve, a big inflammatory response can occur. This inflammatory response makes it hard for damaged axons to regenerate and may bring about confined healing.

Although regenerative plasticity is most normally visible in peripheral nerves, it's far vital to word that the identical degree of regeneration does no longer arise within the applicable worried device, which includes the thoughts and spinal twine. Nerve cells in the essential annoying system have a limited diploma of regenerative capability, which makes injuries to this vicinity greater tough in terms of healing.

The take a look at of regenerative plasticity remains a promising difficulty of studies. Scientists are investigating methods to stimulate and facilitate axonal regeneration in considered one of a type scientific contexts, a terrific manner to enhancing recovery strategies after nerve accidents.

In summary, regenerative plasticity in peripheral nerves is a incredible machine wherein damaged axons can regenerate and regain their function. Although whole regeneration isn't always continuously possible, this phenomenon demonstrates the splendid potential of the disturbing tool to conform and get better after injuries. The have a study of this shape of plasticity continues to beautify, supplying want for future advances within the situation of neurological recuperation.

somatic plasticity

Somatic plasticity refers to our frame's capability to comply and trade in reaction to stimuli and studies. It's like our body has the functionality to form and regulate in keeping with the wishes we are dealing with.

Imagine you're taking up a state-of-the-art game, like tennis. At first, you may have hassle hitting the ball and coordinating your movements. However, as you still exercise, your frame will begin to adapt. Your muscular tissues get stronger, your reflexes grow to be quicker, and you start to enhance your endeavor capabilities. This is an instance of somatic plasticity.

This adaptability is not genuinely constrained to bodily activities, but can rise up in distinctive areas as nicely. For instance, in case you are learning to play a musical device, your mind adjusts and develops particular neural connections related to song. Over time, you emerge as more professional and capable of play greater complex melodies.

Somatic plasticity is present in any respect degrees of existence. That's why children have an terrific capability to research new abilties like speakme, taking walks and writing. Their our our our bodies are constantly adapting and shaping consistent with the critiques and stimuli they get maintain of.

This capacity to exchange and adapt is one of the maximum wonderful matters approximately our our bodies. It permits us to analyze, boom and boom throughout our lives. Somatic plasticity indicates that our body is not a difficult and fast shape, however as an opportunity a malleable entity which could modify.

axonal plasticity

Axon plasticity refers to the capability of axons, the elongated extensions of neurons, to conform and trade in response to stimuli and enjoy. It's as even though axons have the functionality to transform themselves and installation new connections with one-of-a-kind neurons.

Axons are accountable for transmitting electric and chemical signs among neurons, allowing efficient verbal exchange inside the mind and nervous gadget. Axonal plasticity allows the ones connections to be changed, reinforced or maybe created to conform to new conditions and desires.

An instance of axonal plasticity is what takes place within the direction of the gaining knowledge of approach. When we've got a take a look at some component new, like gambling a musical device or speakme a new language, the connections maximum of the axons of the neurons involved in that unique skill are bolstered. This takes place via structural adjustments in axons and synapses, the junctions among neurons that permit signals to be transmitted.

Furthermore, axonal plasticity also plays an essential role in restoration after nerve injuries. When an axon is injured, the axon itself can attempt to regenerate and rebuild misplaced connections. This can also additionally need to incorporate growing new axons or seeking out opportunity routes to hook up with other neurons. This axonal plasticity is essential for beneficial restoration after injuries to the concerned tool.

It is vital to awareness on that axonal plasticity does no longer get up indiscriminately. It is regulated through the use of various of things, which incorporates signaling molecules, genes, and the electric hobby of neurons. Furthermore, axonal plasticity may be influenced by way of the use of environmental elements which incorporates sensory stimuli, gaining knowledge of stories or even the usage of sure drugs.

dendritic plasticity

Dendrites are the small branches of neurons, fundamental structures for receiving nerve stimuli. The greater extensions emerged from the neurons, the extra the neuroplasticity.

The quantity of connections long-established shows the boom in information, integration of information and new reflections regarding a neural feature that changed into out of place in a massive lesion.

Sinapses the Hebb

Hebb synapses are an vital concept in neuroscience that describe how connections among neurons are reinforced based totally mostly on coordinated neuronal hobby. This concept become proposed thru psychologist Donald Hebb in 1949 and is called "Hebb's rule".

According to Hebb's rule, whilst a neuron over and over "fires" and stimulates any other neuron, the synapse among them is strengthened. In simple phrases, the concept is that "neurons that hearth collectively, twine together."

This way that once neurons are active at the identical time, the synapse among them is bolstered. This reinforcement happens thru biochemical mechanisms that lead to physical changes inside the synapses, making them extra inexperienced in transmitting indicators.

Hebb's rule is one of the important concepts of synaptic plasticity, this is, the capability of synapses to alternate in reaction to neuronal interest. It is considered an critical theoretical foundation for facts how analyzing and memory formation stand up within the mind.

When applied in a broader context, Hebb's rule indicates that repeated and coordinated reports among stimuli and responses can purpose the strengthening of corresponding synaptic connections. This manner that analyzing and memory formation rely on the coordinated activation of businesses of neurons that are worried within the equal task or revel in.

However, it is crucial to emphasise that Hebb's rule is simplest one in each of numerous forms of synaptic plasticity. There are exclusive plasticity mechanisms that also play crucial roles in the formation and change of synapses.

They are a idea that describes how synapses between neurons are strengthened based totally on coordinated neuronal hobby. This essential concept, known as Hebb's rule, plays a treasured function in synaptic plasticity and in expertise learning and memory strategies inside the mind.

The female who studied Albert Einstein's thoughts

Marian have become born in 1926 and became a famend neuroscientist in the United States.

In 1984, after the dying of Albert Einstein in 1955, the well-known scientist's thoughts have become preserved for similarly look at. Marian Diamond had the unique possibility to investigate Einstein's thoughts and have a look at whether or not or not there were any precise developments that might explain his genius.

Marian grow to be a pioneer in the area of neuroplasticity, the look at of the thoughts's functionality to conform and exchange for the duration of life. She turned into specially interested in information how environment and way of life might also have an impact on brain form and feature.

By studying Einstein's thoughts, Marian made wonderful discoveries. She referred to that Einstein's mind had a slightly wonderful form in evaluation to the brains of everyday human beings. Specifically, the region known as the prefrontal cortex, that is related to higher cognitive talents like precis thinking and problem fixing, became thicker and denser in Einstein.

This discovery recommended that Einstein's genius may be related to his specific thoughts form. However, it's far essential to word that the connection among mind anatomy and intelligence remains the hassle of take a look at and debate inside the clinical network.

Marian Diamond persevered her career committed to research and training. She has made extensive contributions to the world of neuroscience, advancing records of the significance of environment and way of life in thoughts fitness.

The tale of the lady who studied Albert Einstein's thoughts indicates us how technology can provide us with valuable insights into the complexity of the human mind. Marian Diamond had the particular possibility to discover the secrets and techniques of the mind of definitely certainly one of statistics's greatest geniuses, and her discoveries have contributed to our expertise of mind shape and characteristic.

Chapter 15: The Cool Science Of Brain Change

Hello there, explorer! It's time to begin our exceptional journey. Today we're diving into the thrilling international of Neuroplasticity! You might be wondering, "What inside the global is that? It seems like a huge, horrifying monster!" Well, do not worry, it's far no longer a monster, however it's far big in terms of the way vital it is. And with the aid of the usage of the stop of this financial ruin, you may be a seasoned at information this large phrase or even explaining it to others.

Let's start with a few component a laugh. Picture a large, squishy ball of play-dough. It's easy, bendy, and expecting your creativity to turn it into a few factor amazing. With a chunk of creativeness, you can mildew it right into a race automobile, a cute doggy, a flower, or possibly a dinosaur! And the first-class detail? If you do now not like what you have made, you may truely squish it all again collectively and begin over.

Guess what? Your mind is just like that play-dough! It has the functionality to trade and adapt based totally definitely mostly on new belongings you have a look at and studies you have. This fantastic ability of the mind to reshape and reorganize itself is what we name Neuroplasticity.

Now, permit's destroy down that big, fancy word. 'Neuro' is from neuron, that is just a fantastic medical way to say 'mind mobile.' And 'plasticity?' That comes from 'plastic,' which right right here way able to being molded or customary. So, Neuroplasticity is the mind's capacity to change and reshape itself, much like our play-dough!

Why is that this important? Well, think about at the same time as you first located to journey a bike. It grow to be quite difficult, right? You probably wobbled, fell over a couple of instances, and possibly even favored to surrender. But you saved trying. And bet what? Each time you attempted, your thoughts become converting. It have end up developing new connections and pathways that will help you balance, pedal, and steer. The greater you practiced, the higher you have got come to be, till ultimately, you have got been zipping round like a seasoned! This is Neuroplasticity in movement!

Now, permit's pay interest a story about Tommy, a chunk boy who wasn't exceptional at spelling. He'd aggregate up letters, neglect approximately the proper order, and get virtually annoyed. But Tommy end up a fighter. He began running toward each day, the usage of flashcards, writing in a spelling ebook, or maybe making up a laugh songs approximately complex phrases. Over time, his spelling commenced out to decorate. This did no longer occur via magic, however through Neuroplasticity. His mind modified into converting and developing new pathways that helped him keep in thoughts the right spellings. Cool, isn't it?

But Neuroplasticity isn't pretty lots studying new talents. It can also help our brains get over injuries. Meet Lucy, a extra younger lady who had an accident and harm her thoughts. After the accident, Lucy had hassle transferring her left hand. But she did no longer give up. She practiced each day and wager what? She began getting higher! Even notwithstanding the truth that a few elements of her thoughts were harm, one in all a kind components changed and helped her circulate her hand another time. It's like if a avenue is blocked, you find out a particular direction to your excursion spot. That's precisely what Lucy's thoughts did. And it is the energy of Neuroplasticity!

So, my courageous explorer, aren't our brains remarkable? They have this superpower to observe, adapt, or even heal! They're like our very private superheroes, working tirelessly to assist us get higher at topics and triumph over disturbing conditions.

By now, you're officially a step closer to becoming a Neuroplasticity pro. Our journey has truly commenced out and there's masses extra to find out approximately this wonderful superpower in our brains. Let's get prepared to free up all the outstanding subjects we are capable of do with Neuroplasticity! Stay tuned, explorer!

Chapter 16: Unleashing Potential

Howdy, fellow explorer! Welcome lower back to our adventure through the thrilling world of neuroplasticity! After our first forestall wherein we placed what neuroplasticity is and how it can help us take a look at and heal, it's time to unencumber even extra approximately this captivating problem. Ready to dive deeper and discover about the superpowers hidden inside your thoughts? Let's bypass!

Remember whilst we mentioned our brains being like play-dough? Not absolutely because of the truth they're smooth and squishy, however due to the truth they will be reshaped and modified? Well, this time let's imagine our thoughts is type of a superhero. Now, each superhero has their private precise abilities or powers, right? Just like that, your thoughts additionally has superpowers, way to neuroplasticity!

So, what exactly are those superpowers? Let's find out!

First up, we've the superpower of Learning. Remember when you first determined to tie your shoelaces, revel in a motorcycle, or play a musical instrument? At first, it have become truly tough, wasn't it? But with a touch time and workout, it have emerge as a bit of cake. That's due to the reality your mind created new pathways that will help you study those capabilities. This is your mind's superpower of mastering in motion!

Next is the superpower of Recovery. Let's communicate approximately our friend Lucy from Chapter 1. After her twist of destiny, Lucy had hassle transferring her hand. But with practice and determination, Lucy began out getting better. This is because of the fact her thoughts become capable of reroute and create new pathways, supporting her hand circulate once more. Now, that's what we call the superpower of restoration!

Another great superpower of your mind is Adaptability. This method your thoughts's capability to regulate to new conditions or modifications. Have you ever moved to a brand new region and felt a touch lost? But after a while, you bought used to it, observed new friends, or perhaps located a few cool spots to your community. That's your mind adapting to the brand new surroundings. So, excessive-five for the superpower of adaptability!

And ultimate, however absolutely now not least, is the superpower of Changing Habits. Yes, you heard that right! Your mind will assist you to spoil antique conduct and form new ones. Remember Sam from our preceding communication? He have become gambling video video games too much. But with the assist of his brain's superpower, he turned into capable of create new conduct and find a more healthful stability.

Now, knowing about those superpowers is one factor, however the utilization of them is wherein the real fun begins! Just like a superhero has to discover ways to use their powers, we moreover want to understand a way to unharness those superb abilties of our brains. And don't worry, we are going to do simply that in our upcoming chapters.

As we hold our adventure, we are going to discover a way to harness the ones superpowers to change conduct, growth highbrow flexibility, and even regulate memories! We will see how those superpowers can assist us emerge as higher novices, greater adaptable people, and regular superheroes in our very personal lives.

So, keep tight as we prepare to disencumber the actual functionality of our brains. It's going to be an exciting ride!

Chapter 17: How Brain Change Helps Alter Habits

Hello, courageous explorer! Welcome lower lower returned! We've already located a few terrific subjects on our journey, haven't we? Now, it's time to zoom in on how neuroplasticity can help us trade our conduct. Sound cool? Alright, allow's skip!

You undergo in mind our friend Sam, right? He cherished gambling video video video video games a lot that he might neglect to do his homework. Now, playing video video games isn't lousy in any respect. But forgetting approximately homework and different important topics for it? Not so top. Sam desired to alternate this dependancy, however it turned into clearly hard for him.

Why are behavior so hard to break? Well, conduct, whether or no longer they are actual or terrible, are like nicely-trodden paths in our mind. Think about a course in a park. The greater humans stroll on it, the clearer and additional defined the direction becomes.

Habits paintings the equal manner in our mind. The extra we do some component, the stronger that course will become in our mind.

But proper here's where our superhero, neuroplasticity, is to be had in! Neuroplasticity method we are capable of honestly create new paths in our mind! Think of it like building a cutting-edge, greater wholesome route in that park, one that leads us to a beautiful flower lawn in choice to a prickly thorn bush.

That's what Sam needed to do. He desired to create a latest mind direction in which he might notwithstanding the reality that play video video games, however moreover find time for his homework and chores.

And guess what? Sam succeeded! He started placing a timer even as gambling video video video video games. When the timer went off, he might pause the sport and do a piece of his homework or a chore. It changed into tough in the beginning. Sometimes, he felt like giving up. But he remembered that constructing a ultra-current path takes time and effort.

Slowly however in reality, it have end up much less difficult. Sam began out locating it natural to pause his game and do his art work. He had built a modern-day, extra healthful dependancy. And bet who grow to be within the again of all this? Our movie star, neuroplasticity!

Creating new behavior can be hard earlier than the whole lot. It's much like the ground is all tough and rocky at the same time as we start building a latest course. But with time, staying power, and repetition, we can make that direction easy and smooth to stroll on. And the splendid element? We have our thoughts's superpower, neuroplasticity, to help us alongside the manner!

Chapter 18: Building A More Flexible Mind

Hey there, remarkable explorer! We've been on a quite brilliant journey up to now, have now not we? Today, we are going to step into the thoughts gym to work out our neurons and construct a extra flexible thoughts. Are you ready? Grab your brain footwear and permit's skip!

Did your thoughts is shape of a wonderful-bendy gymnast? Seriously! Just like a gymnast's body can bend and flex, your mind also can stretch and trade. This flexibility of your mind is every unique one of these superpowers we stated. Cool, right?

But proper right here's the aspect: similar to a gymnast wants to train to live bendy, our mind needs its very very very own shape of exercise too. And that's what we're going to talk approximately nowadays.

You is probably thinking, "But how do I schooling consultation my thoughts?" Great query! Let's discover with the resource of visiting our buddy Maria.

Maria likes to treatment puzzles. One day, she found a genuinely tough puzzle. She attempted to solve it, but it emerge as simply too difficult. Maria felt stuck. But then she remembered a few issue her trainer had said approximately the mind's superpower of pliability. So, Maria determined to try a tremendous technique. Instead of searching on the puzzle as a whole, she broke it down into smaller factors. Suddenly, the puzzle failed to appear so frightening. And guess what? Maria solved the puzzle!

That's what mind flexibility is all about - finding new techniques to remedy issues. Just like Maria, we are able to all train our brains to be extra bendy.

But how are we able to try this? Here are a few smooth bodily video video games for our thoughts health club:

1. Try New Things: Doing some issue new, like reading a musical device or a brand new task, can help your thoughts assemble new connections. It's like including new device for your mind health club!

2. Challenge Your Brain: Puzzles, riddles, and thoughts video video games are great exercising workouts on your mind. They help stretch your thoughts's flexibility muscle mass.

3. Be Curious: Asking questions and being curious about the arena round you is some other extremely good manner to exercise your mind. It's like doing brain yoga!

four. Stay Positive: Having a excessive top notch thoughts-set can help your thoughts stay bendy. It's like giving your brain a pep talk in advance than a huge exercise!

five. Rest and Relax: Just like a high-quality workout goals a cool-down, your mind moreover dreams time to rest and lighten up. Good sleep, meditation, or simply quiet time can assist your thoughts get higher and broaden stronger.

Remember, schooling our brains is like education our our our bodies. It takes time and exercising. But with a touch staying power and consistency, we are able to assemble a extra flexible and stronger thoughts.

So, explorer, are you prepared to step into the thoughts gym and stretch your neurons? Remember, your mind's superpower of flexibleness is there to help you. And who is   . aware of? You would possibly likely actually discover that your mind is the extremely good gymnast you realise!

Up subsequent, we are going to examine how our mind can help us save you procrastination. So, stick round, there's extra to find out in our interesting journey!

Chapter 19: Using Brain Science To Stop Procrastination

Hey there, thoughts explorer! Are you prepared for every different interesting bankruptcy in our adventure? Today, we're going to use the superpowers of our thoughts to address a elaborate villain known as Procrastination. I wager we've all met this villain in some unspecified time in the destiny. So, permit's determine out how we can use thoughts technological know-how to say goodbye to geared up and prevent procrastination.

Do you recollect our pal Sam? Yes, the handiest who loved gambling video video video games and had learned to assemble new conduct. Well, Sam had some other mission to stand. He had a big technological records undertaking due, but he saved setting it off. Every time he belief of strolling on it, he placed some thing else to do. Playing video video video games, looking TV, even cleansing his room! Sam end up below the spell of the procrastination villain.

But guess what? Sam has his superhero, neuroplasticity, via manner of his element! And together, they could defeat procrastination.

Let's take a minute to understand our villain. Procrastination takes location whilst our brain chooses some component that makes us satisfied right now over a few detail at the manner to assist us within the future. It's like choosing a sweet bar over a wholesome salad. The candy bar is tempting and makes us happy proper away. But in the long run, the salad is better for us.

So how can Sam use neuroplasticity to conquer procrastination? The answer is an awful lot much less hard than you agree with you studied: he can construct a modern day mind path!

Remember the thoughts fitness center we stated? The sports activities we do there can help us gather new paths. Here's how Sam did it:

1. Break It Down: Sam's generation assignment appeared massive and horrifying. So, he broke it down into smaller, more practicable components, much like he could spoil down a huge puzzle. This made the assignment enjoy a great deal much less overwhelming, and plenty much less tough to begin.

2. One Step at a Time: Instead of seeking to do everything proper away, Sam determined to focus on one small a part of the challenge at a time. This manner, he felt lots tons less confused and will do a better task on each aspect.

3. Reward Time: Every time Sam completed part of his task, he rewarded himself with a quick online game damage. This made his brain satisfied and helped him live encouraged to maintain going.

4. Stay Positive: Even whilst matters were given difficult, Sam attempted to live superb. He knowledgeable himself, "I can do that!" And guess what? His brain believed him!

By doing the ones carrying sports, Sam modified into training his mind to choose out out the technological understanding challenge (the salad) over procrastination (the sweet bar). And the more he practiced, the more potent this new thoughts direction have emerge as.

And guess what? Sam finished his technological know-how undertaking! He felt absolutely thrilled with himself. And the procrastination villain? Well, allow's without a doubt say it failed to stand a risk within the course of Sam and his thoughts's superpower!

Just like Sam, each person can use brain technological recognize-how to forestall procrastination. Remember, it is probably tough at the begin. But with endurance, practice, and our superhero, neuroplasticity, we will assemble a current mind route and defeat the procrastination villain!

Are you geared up for the following part of our journey, in which we're going to discover ways to use our mind to adjust memories?

Buckle up, explorer. We've were given more exciting things to find out!

Chapter 20: How Our Brain Can Change Our Past

Hello all over again, courageous thoughts explorer! Ready to find more thoughts superpowers? Today, we are diving into a part of our mind adventure that might appear a piece like magic. But accept as true with me, it's miles all technology. We're going to find out about how our thoughts can exchange our beyond – properly, shape of. We're speakme about memory magic!

Let's consider recollections as photos in a photo album. When you test a image, you hold in thoughts what befell, right? But have you ever ever found how the records can change? Maybe in the end, you keep in mind wearing a crimson blouse at your party. But the following day, you are effective it have emerge as blue. That's your reminiscence magic at art work!

Now, allow's introduce our friend Ava. Ava had a memory of her canine, Max, walking away in the park. This memory made Ava enjoy scared and sad. She modified into scared to take Max to the park due to the reality she have grow to be afraid he can also run away once more. But then Ava found out approximately reminiscence magic.

With reminiscence magic, we cannot change what without a doubt took place, but we will exchange how we remember it. Ava couldn't alternate the truth that Max ran away, however she may additionally want to change her emotions approximately that reminiscence.

Here's how Ava used her mind's superpower of neuroplasticity to paintings a few reminiscence magic:

1. Understanding the Memory: First, Ava notion about the reminiscence. She idea approximately what happened, the way it made her experience, and why it made her revel in that manner.

2. Change the Perspective: Next, Ava modified the way she looked at the memory. Instead of

focusing on Max running away, she focused at the element wherein Max came again. This made her feel masses happier!

3. Practice the New Memory: Ava concept about the today's, happier model of her reminiscence over and over yet again. Just like running toward a cutting-edge-day sport or a ultra-modern tune, practising the contemporary reminiscence helped her thoughts assemble a cutting-edge day course.

four. Reward the Change: Each time she idea about the new version of the reminiscence, Ava rewarded herself with a cope with. This helped her thoughts discover ways to much like the new reminiscence greater than the antique one.

After a while, Ava wasn't scared to take Max to the park anymore. Instead, she felt satisfied because of the fact she remembered the instances on the same time as Max came lower back to her.

And that, explorer, is the energy of reminiscence magic! With it, Ava used her mind's superpower of neuroplasticity to change her past. Well, form of. She couldn't alternate what truly happened, however she may also want to trade how she felt about it.

As we adventure in addition into the wonders of our brains, consider, like Ava, everybody have this power. We all can use reminiscence magic to trade how we consider our past. And who knows? Maybe we are able to even use it to change our future!

So, are you organized to analyze extra approximately your great mind? Then buckle up! Because our next save you is all approximately your future. We're going to find out approximately developing a mind-wholesome future! I can't wait to proportion this next journey with you!

Chapter 21: Practical Magic

Hey there, intrepid mind explorer! We've come a protracted way on our mind journey, have no longer we? From gaining knowledge of about our mind's superpowers to defeating procrastination, we've got were given uncovered a few top notch topics about our thoughts. Now, we are prepared to wrap up our journey with some sensible magic! We're going to research clean steps to rewire our mind.

Remember our pals Sam and Ava? They every used their thoughts's superpower of neuroplasticity to overcome demanding situations and trade their behavior and memories. Now, it's miles your turn!

Before we dive in, permit's maintain in thoughts that rewiring our thoughts is not like flipping a mild switch. It takes time and exercise, just like studying to journey a motorbike or play the piano. But with staying strength, and a piece little little little bit of sensible magic, we're capable of all discover ways to rewire our brains!

Ready to research the steps? Let's get started out!

1. Identify the Change: First, think about what you need to trade. Maybe you want to forestall biting your nails, or begin doing all of your homework proper after college. Whatever it's miles, write it down.

2. Make a Plan: Next, make a plan for a way you will make the exchange. Think approximately the steps you may want to take, and write those down too. Remember Sam's technological understanding challenge? He broke it down into smaller additives to make it extra functionality.

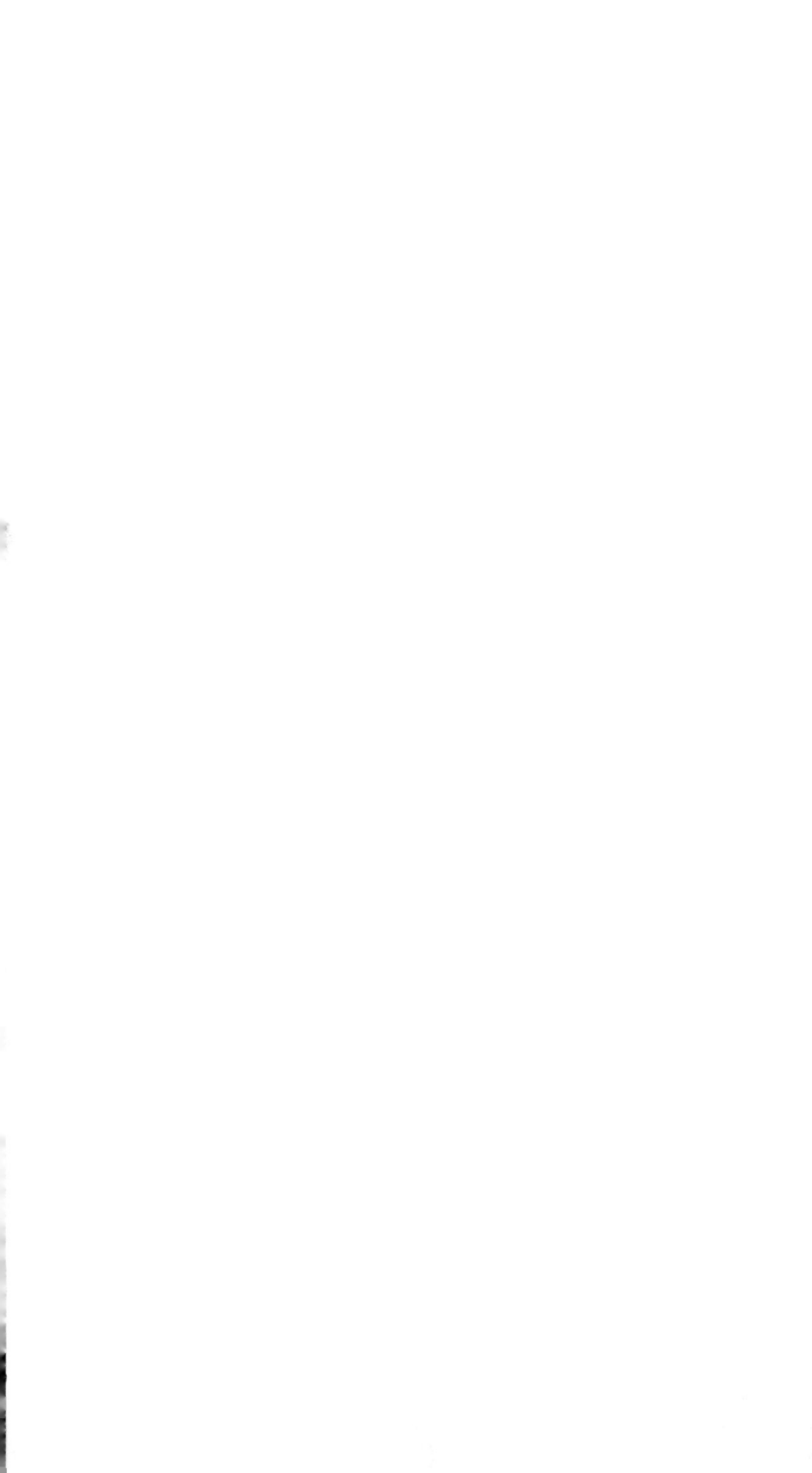

www.ingramcontent.com/pod-product-compliance
Lightning Source LLC
Chambersburg PA
CBHW051727020426
42333CB00014B/1188